CHEST X-RAY

MADE EASY

Jonathan Corne MA PhD MB BS FRCP

Consultant Respiratory Physician, Nottingham University Hospitals NHS Trust, Nottingham, UK

Kate Pointon MRCP FRCR

Consultant Radiologist, Department of Radiology, Nottingham University Hospitals NHS Trust, Nottingham, UK

Foreword by

John Moxham MD FRCP

Professor of Respiratory Medicine; Medical Director
King's College Hospital, London

Third Edition

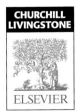

CHURCHILL
LIVINGSTONE

ELSEVIER

Edinburgh   London   New York   Oxford   Philadelphia   St Louis   Sydney   Toronto   2010

CHURCHILL LIVINGSTONE
ELSEVIER

© 2010, Elsevier Limited. All rights reserved.

First Edition 1997
Second Edition 2002
Third Edition 2010

ISBN 978-0-443-06922-2
International ISBN 978-0-443-06735-8

British Library Cataloguing in Publication Data
A catalogue record for this book is available from the British Library

Library of Congress Cataloging in Publication Data
A catalog record for this book is available from the Library of Congress

Notice

Knowledge and best practice in this field are constantly changing. As new research and experience broaden our knowledge, changes in practice, treatment and drug therapy may become necessary or appropriate. Readers are advised to check the most current information provided (i) on procedures featured or (ii) by the manufacturer of each product to be administered, to verify the recommended dose or formula, the method and duration of administration, and contraindications. It is the responsibility of the practitioner, relying on their own experience and knowledge of the patient, to make diagnoses, to determine dosages and the best treatment for each individual patient, and to take all appropriate safety precautions. To the fullest extent of the law, neither the Publisher nor the Authors assumes any liability for any injury and/or damage to persons or property arising out of or related to any use of the material contained in this book.

The Publisher

ELSEVIER your source for books, journals and multimedia in the health sciences

www.elsevierhealth.com

Working together to grow libraries in developing countries

www.elsevier.com | www.bookaid.org | www.sabre.org

ELSEVIER   **BOOK AID** International   Sabre Foundation

The publisher's policy is to use paper manufactured from sustainable forests

Printed in China

Foreword

This short and highly regarded book goes from strength to strength with each edition. Whilst retaining the same basic format, and concentrating on conveying useful advice to junior doctors and clinical medical students, the third edition incorporates important changes. For example, there is more information about chest CT scans. CT scans have now become essential for the management of many patients and it is entirely appropriate that junior staff acquire basic skills in their interpretation. In addition, the CT scans illustrated in this book strengthen the interpretive skills needed to correctly read the chest x-rays.

When I wrote the Foreword for the last edition of this book I commented that clinical decisions affecting the management of patients are often made before the chest x-rays have been formally reported by radiology departments, and the chest x-ray is essentially an extension of the physical examination. This is equally true now. Quality of care, as well as operational efficiency, rely on junior medical staff making the right decisions about the management of their patients as quickly as possible and promptly initiating appropriate therapy. Skills in accurately interpreting the chest x-ray remain as important as ever.

The third edition of *Chest X-ray Made Easy* will, I believe, be highly successful in giving junior doctors the basic skills that they need to correctly interpret chest x-rays, much to the benefit of their patients.

Professor John Moxham,
Professor of Respiratory Medicine; Medical Director,
King's College Hospital,
London

Preface

The chest X-ray is one of the most frequently requested hospital investigations and its initial interpretation is often left to junior doctors. Although there are a large number of specialist radiology textbooks, very few are targeted at junior doctors and medical students. This book was designed to fill this gap and make interpretation of the chest X-ray as simple as possible. It is not meant as an alternative to a radiological opinion but rather as a guide to making sense of the common abnormalities one is likely to encounter on the wards, for speedy recognition of these will expedite effective treatment of the patient.

Following the success of the first and second editions we have expanded the book but still kept it small enough to fit in the pocket. Additional sections have been included and abnormalities under the diaphragm are now discussed. We have also included an introduction to thoracic CT scanning and highlighted the usefulness of these scans where appropriate. The book should remain a useful aid not just for medical students but also for nurses, physiotherapists and radiographers.

Chapters 1 and 2 provide some ground rules that must be applied when interpreting the chest X-ray. Chapter 3 onwards takes the readers through some of the most common abnormalities, arranged according to their X-ray appearance. Each topic contains an example X-ray with an explanatory legend and at the end extra learning points are displayed in the shaded boxes. The outline drawings above the X-rays assist in the interpretation of the abnormality shown.

J.C.
K.P.
2010

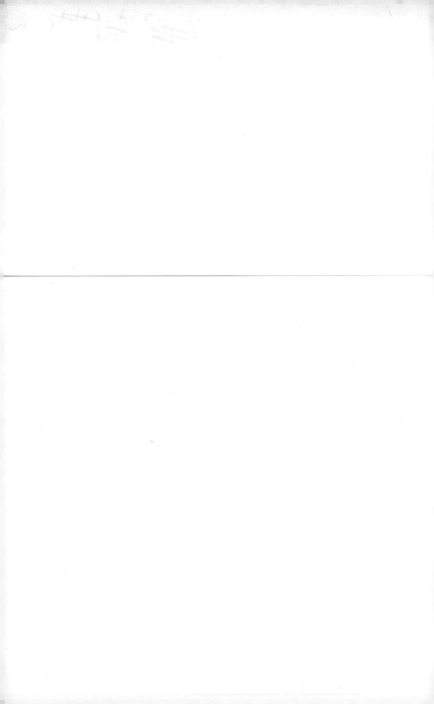

Acknowledgements

We would first like to acknowledge the other co-authors of the first and second edition: Ivan Brown, David Delaney and Mary Carroll. We would also like to acknowledge our colleagues who have read the drafts of this book and made numerous suggestions and contributions, in particular: Kerry Thompson, Fiona Harris, Nicholas Chanarin, Sundeep Salvi, Thirumala Krishna, Peter Hockey, Nicholas Withers, Anoop Chauhan, Mark Bulpitt, Sharon Pimento, Anna McKenzie and Vivienne Okaje. We would like to thank Mary Matteson of the Department of Radiology, Southampton General Hospital for her work in copying the X-rays and the Department of Teaching Media at Southampton General Hospital for producing the final photographs. Kate Pointon would like to thank Lorna Wilson and Maruti Kumaran for their support.

We would also like to thank Professor John Moxham for his invaluable advice with the text and for writing the Foreword, and staff at Elsevier.

Contents

1. How to look at a chest X-ray *1*

1.1 Basic interpretation is easy *2*

1.2 Technical quality *4*

1.3 Scanning the PA film *10*

1.4 How to look at the lateral film *13*

2. Localizing lesions *17*

2.1 The lungs *18*

2.2 The heart *21*

3. The CT scan *27*

4. The white lung field *41*

4.1 Collapse *42*

4.2 Volume loss *54*

4.3 Consolidation *58*

4.4 *Pneumocystis carinii (jiroveci)* pneumonia *62*

4.5 Pleural effusion *64*

4.6 Asbestos plaques *68*

4.7 Mesothelioma *70*

4.8 Pleural disease on a CT scan *72*

Contents

4.9 Lung nodule   *74*

4.10 Cavitating lung lesion   *78*

4.11 Left ventricular failure   *82*

4.12 Acute respiratory distress syndrome   *86*

4.13 Bronchiectasis   *90*

4.14 Fibrosis   *94*

4.15 Chickenpox pneumonia   *100*

4.16 Miliary shadowing   *102*

5. The black lung field   *105*

5.1 Chronic obstructive pulmonary disease   *106*

5.2 Pneumothorax   *110*

5.3 Tension pneumothorax   *112*

5.4 Pulmonary embolus   *114*

5.5 Mastectomy   *119*

6. The abnormal hilum   *121*

6.1 Unilateral hilar enlargement   *122*

6.2 Bilateral hilar enlargement   *126*

7. The abnormal heart shadow   *129*

7.1 Atrial septal defect   *130*

7.2 Mitral stenosis   *132*

7.3 Left ventricular aneurysm   *134*

7.4 Pericardial effusion   *136*

8. The widened mediastinum   *139*

The widened mediastinum   *140*

9. Abnormal ribs *143*

9.1 Rib fractures *144*

9.2 Metastatic deposits *146*

10. Abnormal soft tissues *149*

Surgical emphysema *150*

11. The hidden abnormality *153*

11.1 Pancoast's tumour *154*

11.2 Hiatus hernia *156*

11.3 Air under the diaphragm *158*

Index *161*

CHAPTER 1

How to look at a chest X-ray

1.1 Basic interpretation is
easy 2

1.2 Technical quality. 4

1.3 Scanning the PA film. 10

1.4 How to look at the
lateral film 13

1.1 Basic interpretation is easy

Basic interpretation of the chest X-ray is easy. It is simply a black and white film and any abnormalities can be classified into:

1. Too white.

2. Too black.

3. Too large.

4. In the wrong place.

To gain the most information from an X-ray, and avoid inevitable panic when you see an abnormality, adopt the following procedure:

1. Check the name and the date.

2. If you are using a picture-archiving system, see whether previous X-rays are on the system for comparison. The patient may have had previous X-rays which are stored on film. If you cannot access previous films, look for old radiology reports, which may be helpful.

3. Check the technical quality of the film. (Explained in Chapter 1.2.)

4. Scan the film thoroughly and mentally list any abnormalities you find. Always complete this stage. The temptation is to stop when you find the first abnormality but, if you do this you may get so engrossed in determining what it is that you will forget to look at the rest of the film. Chapter 1.3 explains how to scan a film.

5. When you have found the abnormalities, work out where they are. Decide whether the lesion is in the chest wall, pleura, within the lung or mediastinum. Chapter 2 explains how to localize lesions within the lung and the heart, Chapter 8 the mediastinum and Chapter 9 the ribs.

6. Mentally describe the abnormality. Which category does it fall into:
  I.   Too white.
  II. Too black.
  III. Too large.
  IV. In the wrong place.

Chapters 4 to 11 will take you through how to interpret your findings.

7. Always ensure that the film is reported on by a radiologist. Basic interpretation of the chest X-ray is easy, but more subtle signs require the trained eye of a radiologist. Seeking a radiologist's opinion can often expedite a diagnosis or the radiologist may suggest further imaging.

8. Finally, do not forget the patient. It is possible and, indeed, quite common for a very sick patient to have a normal chest X-ray.

1.2 Technical quality

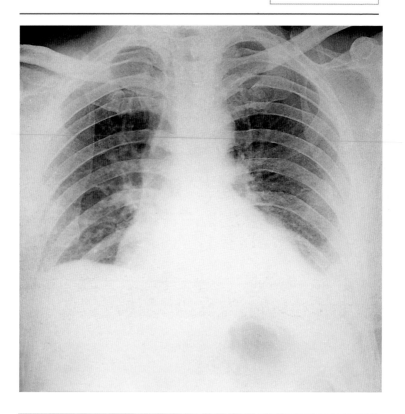

The next four X-rays are examples of how the technical quality of a film can affect its appearance and potentially lead to misinterpretation. Above is an AP film which shows how the scapulae are projected over the thorax and the heart appears large. Compare this to the film opposite which is a standard PA projection showing how the scapulae no longer overlie the thorax and the heart size now appears normal.

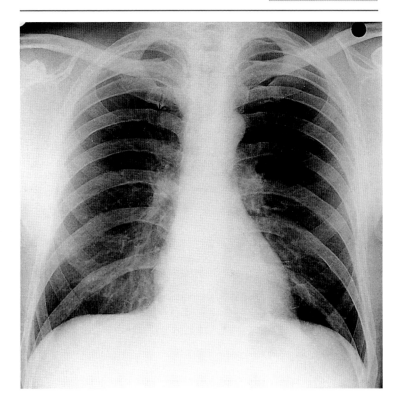

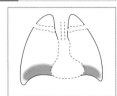

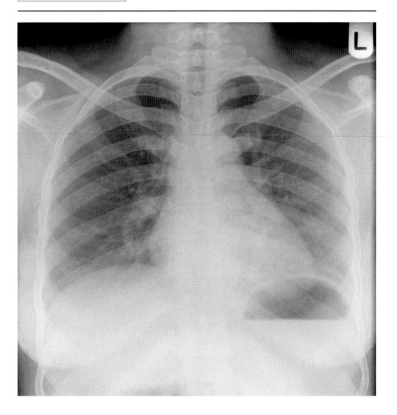

Films on pages 6 and 7 show the effects of respiration. The above film is taken with a poor inspiration, and page 7 with a good inspiration. Note how the lung bases look whiter, and the heart size appears larger.

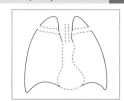

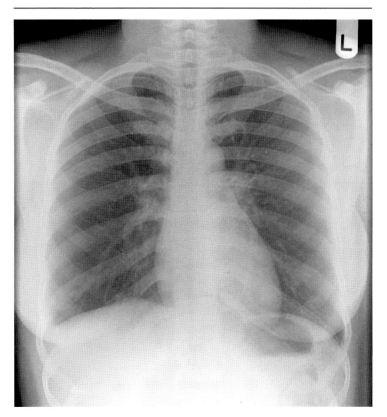

Always check the technical quality of any film before interpreting it further. To do this you need to examine in turn the projection, orientation, rotation, penetration and degree of inspiration. Problems with any of these can make interpretation difficult and unless you check the technical quality carefully you may misinterpret the film.

Projection

Look to see if the film is anteroposterior (AP) or posteroanterior (PA). The projection is defined by the direction of the X-ray beam in relation to the patient. In an AP X-ray the X-ray machine is in front of the patient and the X-ray film at the back. In a PA film the beam is fired from behind the patient and the film placed in front. The standard chest X-ray is PA but many emergency X-rays are AP because these can be taken more easily with the patient in bed. AP films are marked AP by the radiographer and PA films are often not marked since this is the standard projection. If you are not sure then look at the scapulae. If the scapulae overlie the lung fields then the film is AP. If they do not it is most likely PA. If the X-ray is AP you need to be cautious about interpretation of the heart size which will appear magnified on an AP film because the heart is anterior. The shape of the mediastinum can also be distorted. An AP film can be taken with the patient sitting or lying. The film should be marked erect or supine by the radiographer. It is important to note this since the appearance of a supine X-ray can be very different to that of an erect one.

Orientation

Check the left/right markings. Do not assume that the heart is always on the left. Dextrocardia is a possibility but more commonly the mediastinum can be pushed or pulled to the right by lung pathology. Radiographers always safeguard against this by marking the film left and right. Always check these markings when you first look at the film but remember the radiographer can sometimes make mistakes – if there is any doubt re-examine the patient.

Rotation

Identify the medial ends of the clavicles and select one of the vertebral spinous processes that falls between them. The medial ends of the clavicles should be equidistant from the spinous process. If one clavicle is nearer than the other then the patient is rotated and the lung on that side will appear whiter.

A patient with a thoracic scoliosis may appear to have a rotated film. Check whether the spinous processes on the vertebral column are aligned. If they are it is more likely that the patient is rotated.

Penetration

To check the penetration, look at the lower part of the cardiac shadow. The vertebral bodies should only just be visible through the cardiac shadow at this point. If they are too clearly visible then the film is over penetrated and you may miss low-density lesions. If you cannot see them at all then the film is under penetrated and the lung fields will appear falsely white. When comparing X-rays it is important to check that the level of penetration is similar.

Degree of inspiration

To judge the degree of inspiration, count the number of ribs above the diaphragm. The midpoint of the right hemidiaphragm should be between the 5th and 7th ribs anteriorly. The anterior end of the 6th rib should be above the diaphragm as should the posterior end of the 10th rib. If more ribs are visible the patient is hyperinflated. If fewer are visible the patient has not managed a full intake of breath, perhaps due to pain, exhaustion or disease. It is important to note this, as a poor inspiration will make the heart look larger, give the appearance of basal shadowing and cause the trachea to appear deviated to the right. Remember also that patients are all different shapes! Some are broad with relatively short chests and some are tall with long chests. To assess whether the patient has failed to take a deep breath in or simply has a short chest it can be useful to compare the current X-ray with previous ones. If the number of ribs above the diaphragm has changed then it is likely to be due to changes in the degree of inspiration.

1.3 Scanning the PA film

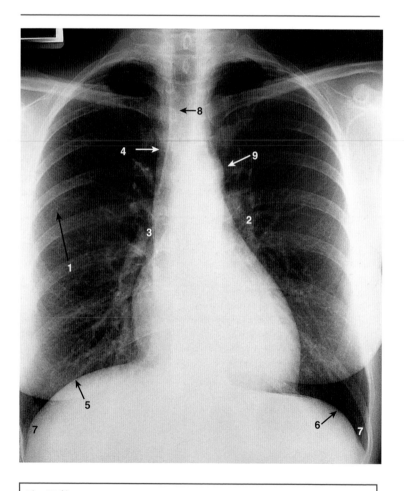

The PA film

If you are looking at a printed film find a decent viewing box with a functioning light that does not flicker. If possible lower the ambient lighting.

If you are using a workstation or computer screen the amount you will see will depend on the resolution of the screen. Make sure you are using a suitable screen and turn down the ambient lighting. You may wish to use an alternative screen if the image is not clear enough. At a workstation the contrast and brightness of the image can be altered to bring out subtle abnormalities; for example, inverting black and white can help make detection of rib abnormalities easier.

If looking at a printed film, in order to recognize areas that are too white or too black you need to survey the X-ray from a distance (about 4 ft/1.2 m) and then repeat this close up.

1. *Lung fields*. These should be of equal transradiancy and one should not be any whiter or darker than the other. Try to identify the horizontal fissure (1) (this may be difficult to see) and check its position. It should run from the hilum to the 6th rib in the axillary line. If it is displaced then this may be a sign of lung collapse.

   An important sign of many lung diseases is loss of volume of that lung and so you need to determine whether either of the lung fields is smaller than it should be. This is difficult since the presence of the heart makes the left lung field smaller. As you see more and more chest X-rays, however, you will gain an appreciation of how the two lung fields should compare in size and therefore be able to detect when one is smaller than it should be.

   Look for any discrete or generalized shadows. These are described in Chapter 4 – The white lung field. Remember that the shadows that appear to be in the lung can represent abnormalities any-where from the patient's clothing and jewellery inwards.

2. *Look at the hilum*. The left hilum (2) should be higher than right (3) although the difference should be less than 2.5 cm. Compare the shape and density of the hila. They should be concave in shape and look similar to each other. Chapter 6 describes how to inter-pret hilar abnormalities.

3. *Look at the heart*. Check that the heart is of a normal shape the maximum diameter is less than half of the trar eter at the broadest part of the chest. Check th abnormally dense areas of the heart shadow. Chap through interpretation of the abnormal heart shad

4. *Check the rest of the mediastinum.* The edge of the mediastinum should be clear although some fuzziness is acceptable at the angle between the heart and the diaphragm. A fuzzy edge to any other part of the mediastinum suggests a problem with the neighbouring lung (either collapse or consolidation) dealt with in Chapter 4. Interpretation of the widened mediastinum is dealt with in Chapter 8.

Look also at the right side of the trachea. The white edge of the trachea (4) should be less than 2–3 mm wide on an *erect* film. (See Chapter 8 for interpretation.)

5. *Look at the diaphragms.* The right diaphragm (5) should be higher than the left (6) and this can be remembered by thinking of the heart pushing the left diaphragm down. The difference should be less than 3 cm. The outline of the diaphragm should be smooth. The highest point of the right diaphragm should be in the middle of the right lung field and the highest point of the left diaphragm slightly more lateral.

6. *Look specifically at the costophrenic angles* (7). They should be well-defined acute angles.

7. *Look at the trachea* (8). This should be central but deviates slightly to the right around the aortic knuckle (9). If the trachea has been shifted it suggests a problem within the mediastinum or pathology within one of the lungs.

8. *Look at the bones.* Step closer to the X-ray and look at the ribs, scapulae and vertebrae. Follow the edges of each individual bone to look for fractures. Look for areas of blackness within each bone and compare the density of the bones which should be the same on both sides. Sometimes turning the image on its side can make rib fractures easier to see.

9. *Soft tissues.* Look for any enlargement of soft tissue areas.

10. *Look at the area under the diaphragm.* Look for air under the diaphragm or obviously dilated loops of bowel. Remember that abdominal pathology can occasionally present with chest symptoms.

1.4 How to look at the lateral film

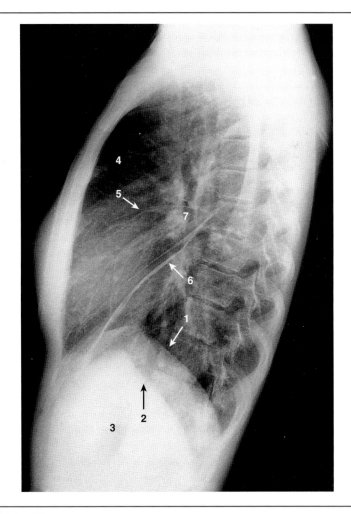

Lateral film

A lateral chest X-ray can be taken with either the right or left side of the patient against the film. Do not worry about which way it has been taken since for all but the most subtle signs it makes little difference. It is useful to get into the habit of always looking at the film the same way and we suggest looking at the film with the vertebral column on the right and the front of the chest on the left. Once you have done this:

1. Check the name and the date.

2. Identify the diaphragms. The right hemidiaphragm (1) can be seen to stretch across the whole thorax and can be clearly seen passing through the heart border. The left (2) seems to disappear when it reaches the posterior border of the heart.

Another method of identifying the diaphragms is to look at the gastric air bubble (3). Look again at the PA film and work out the distance between the gastric air bubble (which falls under the left diaphragm) and the top of the left diaphragm. Make a note of this. Now go back to the lateral. The diaphragm that is the same distance above the gastric air bubble is the left diaphragm.

You can now set about interpreting the film. As with the PA step back from the film and adopt the following process:

1. Compare the appearance of the lung fields in front of and above the heart to those behind. They should be of equal density. Check that there are no discrete lesions in either field.

2. Look carefully at the retrosternal space (4), which should be the blackest part of the film. An anterior mediastinum mass will obliterate this space turning it white.

3. Check the position of the horizontal fissure (5). This is a faint white line which should pass horizontally from the midpoint of the hilum to the anterior chest wall. If the line is not horizontal the fissure is displaced. Check the position of the oblique fissure (6) which should pass obliquely downwards from the T4/T5 vertebrae, through the hilum, ending at the anterior third of the diaphragm.

4. Check the density of the hila (7). A hilar mass may make the hila whiter than usual.

5. Check the appearance of the diaphragms. Occasionally a pleural effusion is more obvious on a lateral film. Its presence would cause a blunting of the costophrenic angle either anteriorly or posteriorly.

6. Look at the vertebral bodies. These should get more translucent (darker) as one moves caudally. Check that they are all the same shape, size and density. Look for collapse of a vertebra or for vertebrae that are significantly lighter or darker than the others, which may indicate bone disease. Consolidation in the posterior costophrenic sulcus can also make the vertebral bodies appear abnormally white.

CHAPTER 2

Localizing lesions

2.1 The lungs 18

2.2 The heart 21

2.1 The lungs

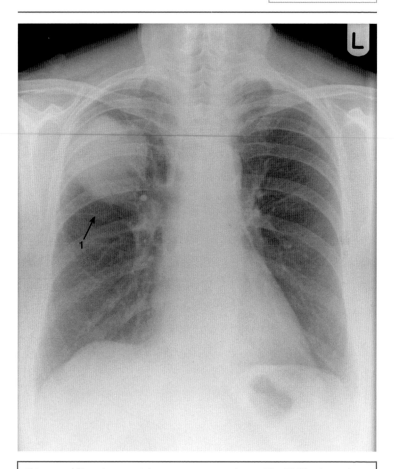

This pair of films shows a right upper zone mass lesion. The PA film shows that it lies above the horizontal fissure (1) and the lateral film that it lies in front of the oblique fissure, as well as above the horizontal fissure (2), so the mass lies in the right upper lobe.

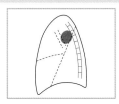

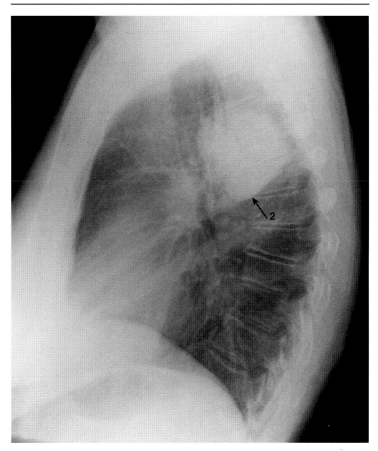

As well as knowing what a lesion is it is often important to know its position within the lung. To accurately localize a lesion on a chest X-ray you need to look at both the PA and lateral films. First look at the PA film:

1. The position of the lesion can be described in terms of zones. The upper zone lies above the right anterior border of the 2nd rib, the middle zone between the right anterior borders of the 2nd and 4th ribs, and the lower zone between the right anterior border of the 4th rib and the diaphragm. Although this is useful descriptively it does not give any information about the lobes of the lung.

2. Look at the borders of the lesion. If the lesion is next to a dense (white) structure then the border between the lesion and that structure will be lost – this is called the silhouette sign. Therefore if the lesion is in the right lung and obscures part of the heart border it must be in the right middle lobe. If it obscures the border of the diaphragm it is in the right lower lobe.

If the lesion is not going to be localized by CT, then a lateral film will be needed.

Using the lateral, if the lesion is in the right lung:

1. Identify the oblique fissure (see p. 14). If the lesion lies posterior to the oblique fissure it must lie within the lower lobe no matter how high it appears on the PA film.

2. If the lesion lies anterior to the oblique fissure it may be in the upper or middle lobe. Identify the horizontal fissure (see p. 14). If the lesion is below the horizontal fissure it is in the middle lobe. If it is above it is in the upper lobe.

If the lesion is in the left lung:

1. Identify the oblique fissure. If it is behind the oblique fissure it must be in the lower lobe. If it is anterior to the oblique fissure it is within the upper lobe – there is no middle lobe on the left!

See Chapter 3, which describes localizing using CT scanning.

2.2 The heart

In order to fully assess any abnormalities of the shape of the heart it is important to understand the composition of the heart shadow. Look at the following four films on pages 22–25.

1. Look at the right heart border and follow it up from the diaphragm. From the diaphragm to the hilum the heart border is formed by the edge of the right atrium (1). From the hilum upwards it is formed by the superior vena cava (2).

2. Follow the left heart border up from the diaphragm. From the diaphragm up to the left hilum it consists of the left ventricle (3). The left border is then concave at the lower level of the left hilum and here it is made up of the left atrial appendage (4). This concavity is lost when the left atrium is enlarged leading to a straightening of the left heart border and sometimes the development of a convexity at this point. At the level of the hilum the border is made up of the pulmonary artery (5) and above this the aortic knuckle (6).

The lateral film is useful. The posterior border of the heart shadow is made up of the left ventricle (7) and the anterior border the right ventricle (8). For example, to identify whether a valve replacement is mitral or aortic, draw an imaginary line from the apex of the heart to the hilum. If the replacement valve lies above this line it is aortic and if it lies below or on, it is mitral.

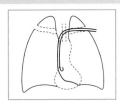

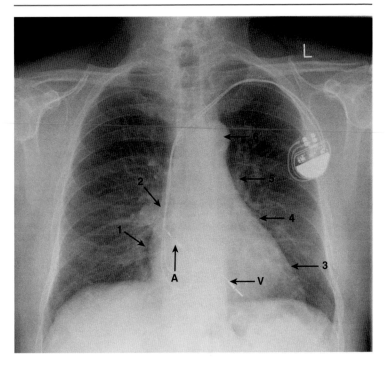

This film is of a patient with an atrial (A) and ventricular (V) pacing wire, with the pacemaker box over the left anterior chest. The atrial wire attaches in the right atrial appendage, and the ventricular wire lies across the tricuspid valve and attaches to the wall of the right ventricle. The numbers are explained in the text on page 21.

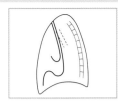

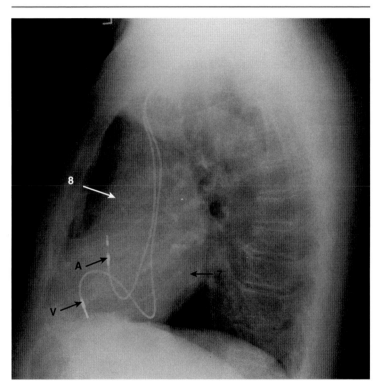

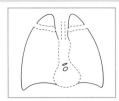

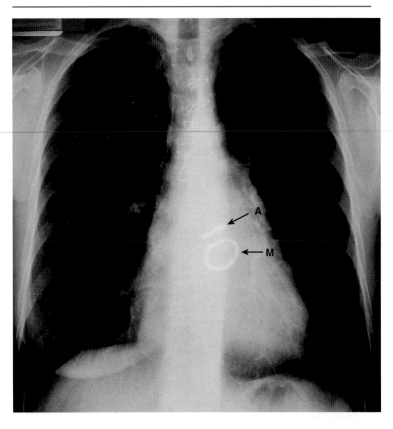

This film is of a patient with prosthetic aortic (A) and mitral (M) valves showing their position in the AP and lateral films.

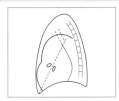

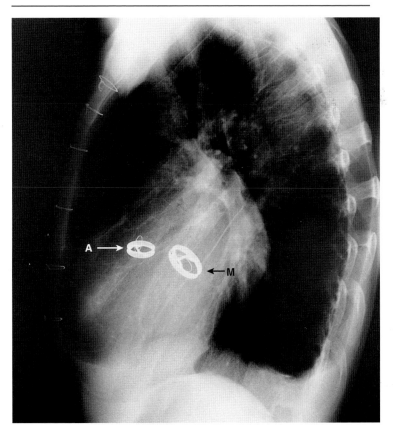

CHAPTER 3

The CT scan

Although the plain chest X-ray is one of the most useful imaging techniques, it is limited by the fact that it is a two-dimensional image and small or subtle abnormalities can be overlooked. In other circumstances the chest X-ray will identify an abnormality but will give limited information as to its extent or detailed appearance. Remember also that, although particularly useful for detecting lung abnormalities, the chest X-ray is a very poor way of imaging the mediastinum.

CT scanning

A CT scanner takes multiple cross-sectional images of the body. A completed CT scan of the chest usually consists of two complete sets of images, one showing mediastinal structures (in which the lung fields look relatively black) and one showing the lung fields in which the mediastinum looks relatively white. These are called the mediastinal and lung windows. These two sets are necessary because there are not enough shades of grey to display adequately both the high-density mediastinal structures and the low-density lungs using one linear scale. In the lung windows the grey scale is expanded across the range of lower density structures, whereas in the mediastinal windows the scale is expanded over the higher-density structures.

Types of CT scan

Two main types of CT scans are performed for the chest: contiguous (spiral) and high resolution. You will need to understand the difference between these in order to know what to request and also to appreciate their limitations. If you include all the relevant history on the scan request, and clearly state the question that needs answering, the radiologist is much more likely to undertake the most appropriate scan.

High-resolution CT scanning (HRCT)

This is a sampling test, which means that not all the lung is examined. With this technique 1–2 mm slices are taken about 10 mm apart. This technique is very good for detecting interstitial lung disease since the thin slices allow for a very detailed assessment of lung architecture (rather like a thin tissue slice enables a pathologist to see more detail). It is not a good technique for finding mass lesions (for example, lung tumours) because the lesion could occur in one of the spaces between the slices and so be missed. The HRCT scan is usually acquired over several breath holds.

Intravenous contrast would not be used with HRCT, since contrast would need to be given before each individual image was taken – something that is clearly impossible.

Spiral CT

This is also called helical CT or volumetric CT. In this technique the anode of the scanner rotates continuously while the table on which the patient lies is moved at a predetermined speed. This technique has the advantage that it is extremely quick – 7 to 10 seconds. The whole chest is scanned, so that small lesions are not likely to be missed, unlike in high-resolution CT where there is a gap between the slices. Sometimes patients are so breathless that they breathe during the scan, causing blurring of the images and making interpretation more difficult.

Spiral CTs are used when intravenous contrast needs to be administered, for example when staging a lung cancer or detecting a pulmonary embolus. The exact timing of the administration of contrast depends on the abnormality being sought. For example, contrast will be injected at a different time for the detection of a pulmonary embolus than it would be if it was being used to enhance the structures of the mediastinum. This is another reason why it is important to be specific about the clinical question being asked when requesting a scan. In addition, this needs to be noted when interpreting scans. For example, a scan performed to stage a lung cancer cannot be used to exclude a pulmonary embolus.

Combined imaging

Many CT scanners are able to acquire spiral images, and with the same data set can process the image to produce a high-resolution study. If a patient only needs a high-resolution CT, this should be requested, as combined imaging exposes the patient to a higher radiation dose.

Interpreting the images

Interpretation of the CT scan requires significant expertise and should only be done by a radiologist. As well as having the experience to interpret the image slices, radiologists have access to software that will allow them to display the images in other forms, for example in the sagittal and coronal planes as well as cross-sectional and three-dimensional images. The CT scans we have included in this book have been chosen because they illustrate situations in which, working on the wards, emergency department or outpatients, you are likely to order scans and a basic knowledge of how they are interpreted will be of use. The next section will give you a basic knowledge of the anatomy of the scan that should help you visualize abnormalities reported on by the radiologist.

Finding your way around the CT scan

It is complicated, but if you learn a few basic areas of anatomy, the rest can be built on later. As with a plain chest X-ray it is important that you have a scheme to work with. Remember, you never look down on a patient, so all CT images are taken as though you are looking up the body from the feet, and the left structures are on the right!

1. Start with the mediastinal windows. Identify the image that shows the arch of the aorta (1) and on this slice:

   a. Look for the trachea, the black circle medial to the arch (2).

   b. Look for the superior vena cava (SVC) (3) which lies to the right of the aorta, and tends to be oval rather than round because the blood is under low pressure.

2. You now need to look at the images above (or cranial) to the one you have just looked at. Make your way up the chest looking at each slice. The lungs will get smaller as you move upwards and the aorta will disappear.

   a. The vessels now visible are the vessels that have come off from the top of the aortic arch. These are the brachio-cephalic artery (4) (this will soon split to form the right subclavian and carotid artery), the left subclavian (5), and the left carotid (6).

   b. There are two further vessels that can be seen, both slightly more anterior than the arteries. These are the left (7) and right (8) brachio-cephalic veins, which will join together to form the SVC that you could see on the first slice you looked at.

3. Now look even higher. You cannot see any lungs because you are now looking above the level of the lung apices. The black hole of the trachea can be seen. Either side of this is a high density (white) structure (9), this is not a blood vessel, but is the thyroid. This is white because it contains iodine, as well as being a very vascular structure. It will appear white even on an unenhanced scan.

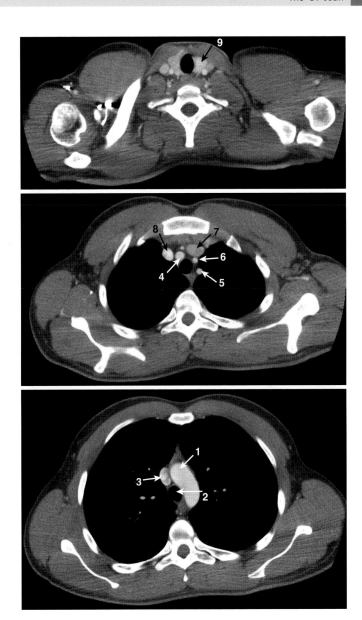

4. Now go back to the original slice, and follow the scans downwards. The lungs will get bigger, and the heart will gradually appear.

a. Now that you are below the level of the arch, the aorta appears twice – the ascending aorta (10), which appears in the middle, and the descending aorta (11), which lies posteriorly.

b. The other white structure is shaped like an inverted Y. This is the pulmonary trunk (12), splitting into the left (13) and right (14) pulmonary arteries. There is no longer a black circle for the trachea, as this has split into the main bronchi and will be better seen on the lung windows later.

c. There is a very small black circle in front of the descending aorta. This is the oesophagus (15), which is sometimes collapsed, or may contain air, as in this case. It is often difficult to see.

5. Move further down. Now you can see the heart.

a. Embryologically the heart was a midline structure that then rotated to the left; this means the left chambers will lie behind the right chambers. The contrast used to enhance the scan lies mainly in the blood pool, so this helps to define the chambers versus the walls of the heart. The thick-walled left ventricle can be seen and is oval in shape (16). The right heart (17) has a much thinner wall and fits around the left ventricle, so it has a more complex outline. Remember to look at the cardiothoracic ratio, since, as with the plain chest X-ray, this should be less than 50% of the bony diameter of the thorax.

b. A few smaller bright areas are seen in the lungs. These are the smaller pulmonary arteries and veins.

6. The lowest image we have given you shows the diaphragm and liver. It is an area that causes a lot of confusion, as the top of the diaphragm can easily be mistaken for a mass.

a. The rounded descending aorta is seen posteriorly (18).

b. There is an area of poorly defined whiteness seen adjacent to the liver/diaphragm. This is the inferior vena cava coming from below to drain blood upwards into the right side of the heart (19).

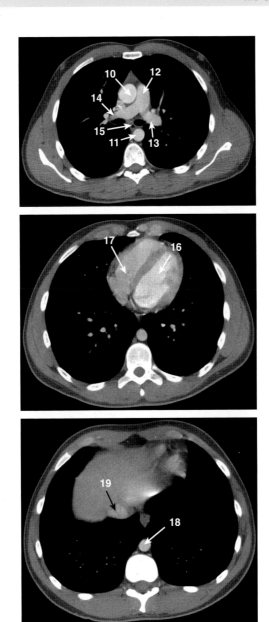

Now look at the lung windows. Start from the top image. You will need to know how to identify the lobes of the lung, so that you can localize any pathology.

1. See images on p. 35 and 36. You will be able to identify the trachea (20). Follow this down until it splits into the left (21) and right (22) main bronchi. Where they split is known as the carina (23).

2. See images on p. 36–38. Identify the main bronchi.

   a. On the right, the right main bronchus splits to give off an oval black tube, the upper lobe bronchus (24). The remaining airway is now called the bronchus intermedius (25). This gives off an anterior branch which is the middle lobe bronchus (26), and the rest continues downwards and backwards as the lower lobe bronchus (27).

   b. See images on p. 36–38. On the left, the upper lobe bronchus gives rise to the airway going to the lingula (28), and the lower lobe bronchus is left by itself (29). It may help to remember that the left lower lobe is smaller than the right because of the space taken by the heart.

3. You can follow the bronchi to identify the main lobes of the lung. The lobes of the lung are surrounded by fissures and you should try to identify these in order to work out the borders of each lobe. The appearance of a fissure will differ depending on the slice thickness. On an HRCT the fissure will appear as a thin white line. On a spiral CT with thicker slices the fine white line is often lost. The blood supply to each lung comes from the hilum, and the vessel branches get smaller as you go to the periphery of the lung, therefore on a thicker slice CT instead of a white line, you see a darker linear strip. No blood vessels are seen to cross the fissure.

   See images on p. 35–38. Identify the major fissures on the left (30) and right (31) and the minor fissure (32) on the right. On the left the major fissure separates the upper and lower lobes. On the right the major fissure separates the lower lobe from the rest of the lung and the minor fissure separates the upper and middle lobes. The minor fissure can be difficult to spot.

4. Now look at the edge of the lungs. You should not be able to see normal pleura, as it is so thin; if there is density here, it must be abnormal.

5. Being able to identify the bronchi is important as it confirms which lobe any pathology lies within, but also remember to look inside the bronchi themselves, as there may be a tumour or an aspirated foreign body.

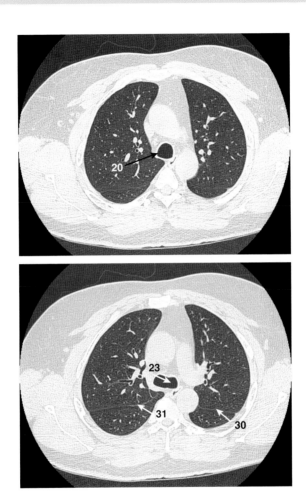

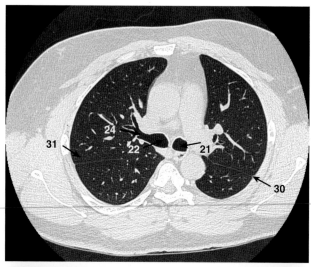

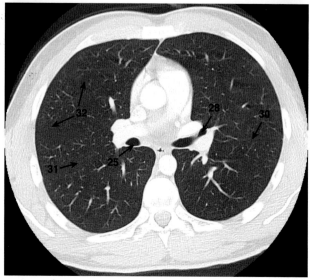

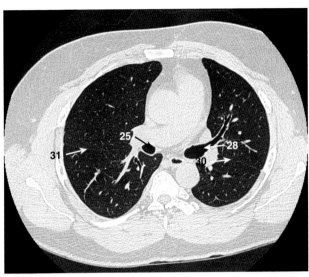

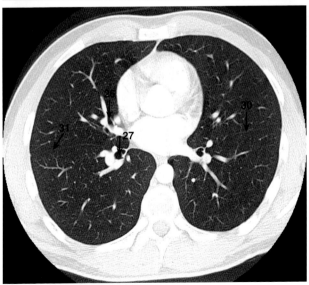

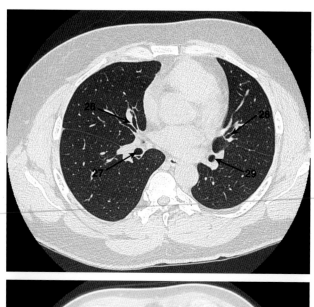

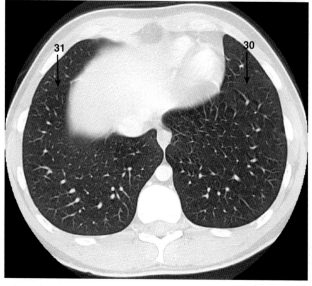

Now that you have identified the normal structures, look for enlarged lymph nodes. You need to distinguish lymph nodes from blood vessels.

1. A lymph node tends to be oval in shape. A blood vessel connects to smaller and larger branches which you will see on several of the adjacent scans, whereas a lymph node is a discrete structure with no connections. When a scan has been contrast enhanced, blood vessels will appear whiter than the lymph nodes and lymph nodes often have central low-density area, as they may contain fat in the middle. An inflamed or malignant lymph node will often be enlarged. We describe lymph nodes, when we see them on a slice at CT, by their shortest not their longest measurement. In the chest a lymph node is considered enlarged if it is more than 10 mm across. The lymph nodes occur in particular places:

   a. Next to the trachea, at many levels.

   b. Underneath the aortic arch.

   c. In front of and beneath the tracheal bifurcation (known as the carina).

   d. At the hila, next to the pulmonary arteries and veins.

2. Look at the bone and soft tissues surrounding the lungs. Check that the surfaces of the bones are continuous, as fractures and metastases need to be considered. Also review the soft tissues; the CT enables you to see the skin and subcutaneous fat as well as muscles.

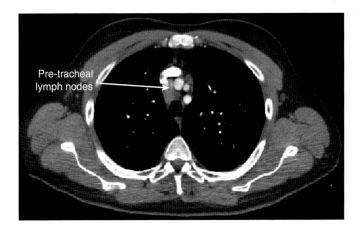

Pre-tracheal lymph nodes

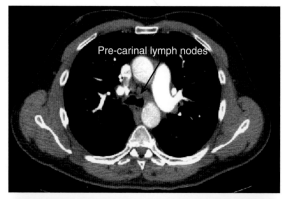

Pre-carinal lymph nodes

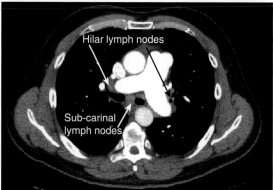

Hilar lymph nodes

Sub-carinal lymph nodes

Artefacts

There are several artefacts that can be seen on the image and can cause confusion. These may be related to patient movement, such as breathing or moving on the table, which causes a blurring of the image. There will also be cardiac motion, which can blur the appearance of the lung closest to the heart.

When contrast is being injected there is very dense fluid flowing through the veins into the right heart. This density, especially when it is in the superior vena cava, causes white streakiness in the adjacent structures. This is called a streak artefact and can sometimes obscure important information. To counter this the radiologist will sometimes wash the contrast out with a second injection of saline. Metalwork such as spinal fixators will also cause significant streak artefact.

CHAPTER 4

The white lung field

4.1 Collapse 42

4.2 Volume loss 54

4.3 Consolidation 58

4.4 *Pneumocystis carinii (jiroveci)*
pneumonia 62

4.5 Pleural effusion 64

4.6 Asbestos plaques 68

4.7 Mesothelioma 70

4.8 Pleural disease on a CT
scan 72

4.9 Lung nodule 74

4.10 Cavitating lung lesion . . . 78

4.11 Left ventricular failure 82

4.12 Acute respiratory distress
syndrome 86

4.13 Bronchiectasis 90

4.14 Fibrosis 94

4.15 Chickenpox pneumonia . . .100

4.16 Miliary shadowing 102

4.1 Collapse

Collapse of a lung is an important cause of a white lung on X-ray. When confronted with a white lung it is important to be thorough in looking for the features suggestive of collapse since the presence of collapse indicates possible serious pathology.

Collapse of the lung leads to a loss of volume of that part of the lung and so the normal radiological landmarks will be distorted. To diagnose collapse look at each of these markings carefully and decide whether they are in the correct position. You may need to look at the lateral X-ray as well as the PA.

On the PA film:

1. If possible, compare with previous films – the change may be long-standing and benign and may not require further investigation. Of course, the clinical context must always be considered.

2. Look at the lung fields. The right lung should be larger than the left – if it is not, suspect an area of right-sided collapse.

3. Look at the diaphragms. The right diaphragm is usually higher than the left. Collapse in the left lung may distort this.

4. Look for the horizontal fissure in the right lung (pp. 18, 19). The horizontal fissure on the right should run from the centre of the right hilum to the level of the 6th rib at the axillary line. If this is pulled up it suggests right upper lobe collapse or, if pulled down, right lower lobe collapse.

5. The heart should straddle the midline with one-third to the right and two-thirds to the left. The heart shadow will be deviated to the side of collapse.

6. The heart borders should be distinct. If the lung adjacent to the heart is collapsed then the heart border will appear blurred. If the right heart border is blurred this indicates right middle lobe collapse and if the left is blurred, lingular collapse.

7. The trachea should be central. Collapse of the right or left upper lobes can pull the trachea towards the area of collapse. Again this may be easier to spot by comparing with the patient's old films.

On the lateral film:

Check the position of the oblique and horizontal fissures (pp. 13 and 14). Any displacement from their normal position suggests collapse. Collapse of any of the lobes of the lung gives a distinct appearance on the X-ray.

Volume loss

A more subtle concept is that of volume loss. Many pulmonary processes, including collapse, may cause progressive amounts of volume change during their evolution. Volume loss will decrease the vascularity of the unaffected part of the lung which will look blacker as a result as this lobe has to over-inflate, so the vessels become more spread out. This is a difficult sign to detect.

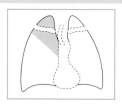

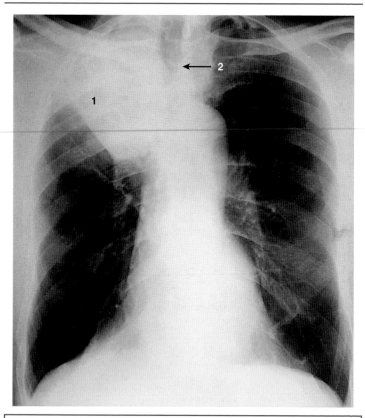

1. **Right upper lobe collapse.** There is an area of whiteness in the upper zone of the right lung (1). The horizontal fissure is elevated, there is an apparent right upper hilar 'mass', the trachea is deviated to the right (2) and the ribs over the area of whiteness are closer together than is normal. On the lateral film the increased whiteness in the uppermost part of the chest may be seen.

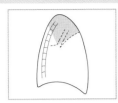

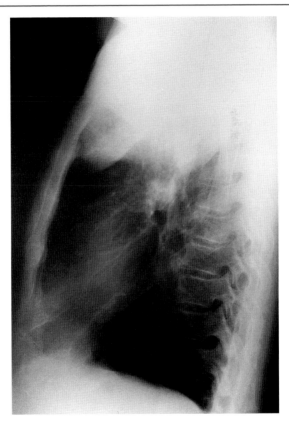

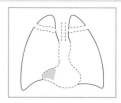

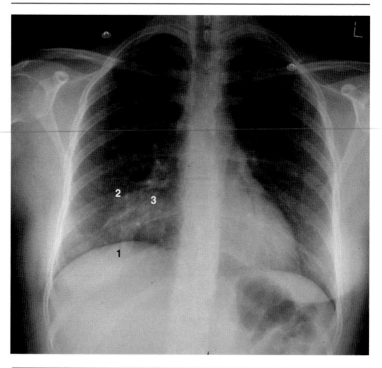

2. **Right middle lobe collapse.** This can be difficult to spot. The right diaphragm may be slightly raised (1) and the horizontal fissure (2) may be
   lower than usual. The upper part of the lower zone may have a hazy white
   appearance (3) and the heart border is sometimes indistinct. It is easier to
   detect in the lateral film. There is a triangular area of whiteness with its
   apex at the hilum (4) and its base running between the sternum and the
   diaphragm (5).

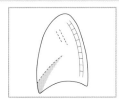

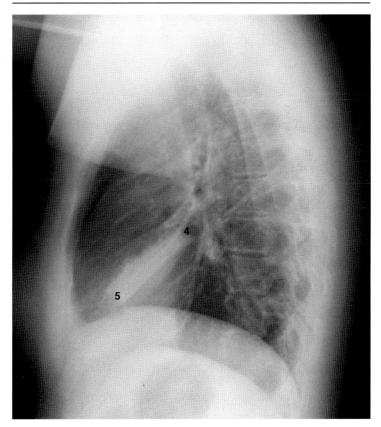

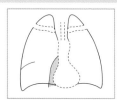

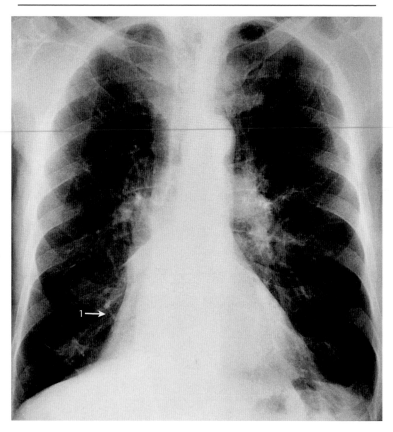

3. **Right lower lobe collapse.** There is a whiteness immediately above the diaphragm (1) causing a loss of its outline. On the lateral film there is a white triangle at the lower posterior part of the lung field (2). Note how the outline of the right heart border is maintained.

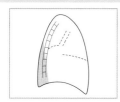

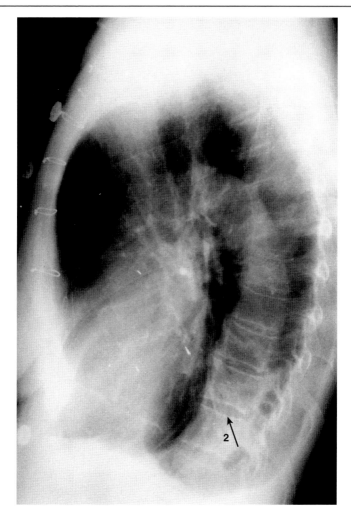

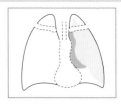

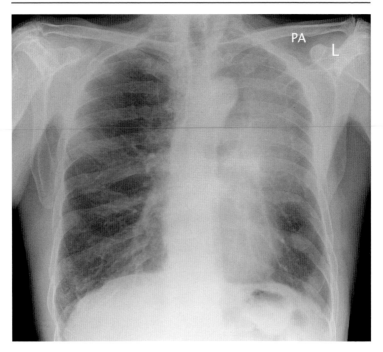

PA

L

---

4. **Left upper lobe collapse.** This is difficult to spot. Remember that most of the left upper lobe lies in front of, as opposed to above, the left lower lobe. When it collapses it causes a haze to appear over the whole of the left lung field.

    The CT image shows the midpoint of the mediastinum shifted to the left (1). The left upper lobe bronchus is filled by a soft tissue density: a tumour. (2). The diagnosis can be easily achieved at bronchoscopy.

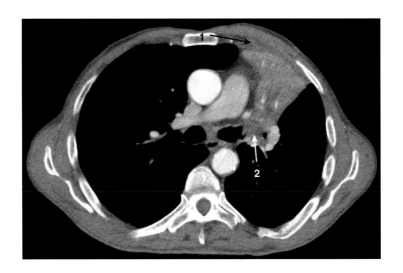

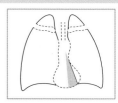

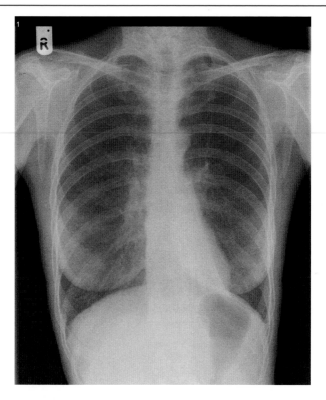

5. Left lower lobe collapse. This is easy to miss. The left lower lobe collapses down behind the heart. The left lung field appears much darker than normal and the heart shadow will appear much whiter than normal. If you look carefully you can see a white triangle behind the heart (1). On the lateral film you may see a white triangle at the bottom posterior corner of the lung fields (2) and the vertebral bodies will appear whiter.

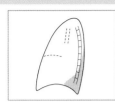

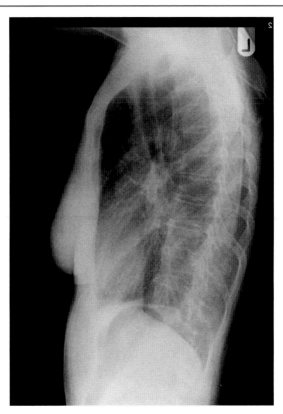

4.2 Volume loss

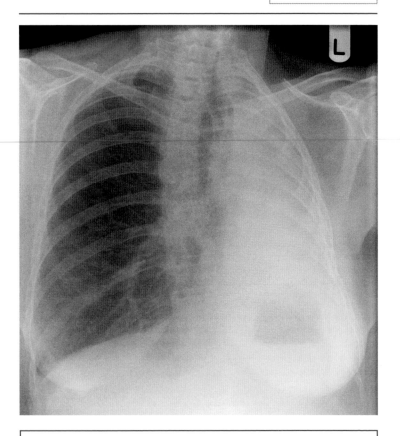

This patient had a pneumonectomy several years ago. The left hemi-thorax is white, and the mediastinum has shifted to the left. The left-sided ribs are also crowded together compared to the right side, and the patient has developed a slight curvature of the spine. The right lung becomes hyperinflated, and some of the lung crosses over the midline.

A pneumonectomy is another cause of a white lung. You should know from the history and your examination that the patient has had a pneumonectomy. Look at the X-ray for the following features:

1. Look at the mediastinum. Look first at the trachea, which should be shifted to the side of the pneumonectomy, then look at the heart border. With a pneumonectomy the heart is often shifted so far that its border is no longer visible.

2. Look at the opposite lung field. Since the mediastinum is shifted the contralateral lung is hyperinflated and so appears darker than usual.

3. Look at the side of the whiteness. You should not be able to see the upper border of the diaphragm on the side of the pneumonectomy.

4. Look carefully at the ribs. If the patient has had a pneumonectomy, ribs would either have been cut or removed during the operation. Therefore look for any rib deformity or note the absence of any rib which would help confirm the diagnosis. The most usual rib to be affected is the 5th.

> A very rare cause of a similar appearance is extensive hypoplasia or congenital absence of one lung.

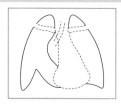

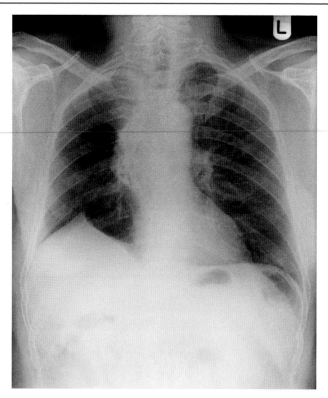

This patient had right upper lobectomy and postoperative radiotherapy. Both of these have led to volume loss in the remaining right lung. The trachea has been pulled to the right as a result. The lung is of increased blackness on the right compared to the left because the remaining lung is hyperinflated.

The right diaphragm has also changed shape, and this appearance is known as diaphragmatic tenting. It looks as though a tent pole has been put underneath to push it upwards.

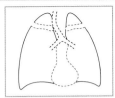

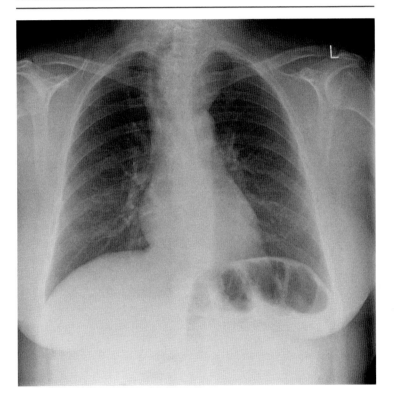

Tracheal deviation can be the result of it being pushed by a mass lesion in the mediastinum, most often an enlarged thyroid gland, as in the case shown here. The lung volumes in this case are normal, and the ribs and diaphragms are in their normal positions. In the elderly a very tortuous aorta may also lead to tracheal shift.

4.3 Consolidation

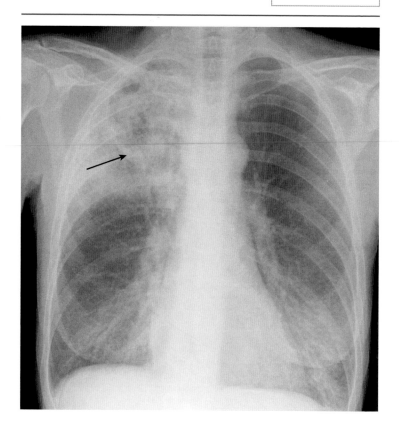

This is the appearance of a lobar pneumonia. Notice how the inferior margin of the consolidation is quite straight. This appearance indicates a right upper lobe pneumonia. An air bronchogram (arrow) is visible.

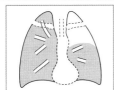

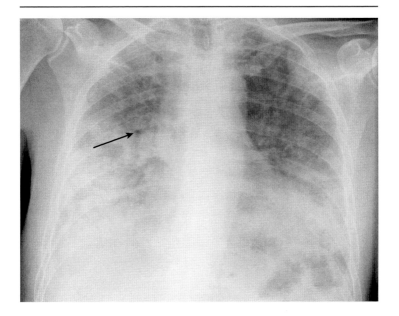

This shows much more widespread consolidation affecting both lungs, especially in the mid to lower zones, and is a bronchopneumonia. An air bronchogram (arrow) is again visible.

Again you can see an area of white lung. Look first at the nature of the whiteness and its border. If it is uniform with a well-demarcated border you are much more likely to be dealing with an area of collapse or a pleural effusion. If the shadowing is not uniform and the border is not so well demarcated the possibilities are consolidation, fibrosis or some other infiltrative condition. It can be difficult to diagnose consolidation so make your way carefully through the following steps:

1. Remember the clinical history. In the presence of a temperature and signs of infection, consolidation is by far the most likely abnormality.

2. Look at old X-rays. Fibrosis is usually a chronic condition and consolidation much more transient. The presence of a similar abnormality on a previous X-ray should lead you to suspect fibrosis rather than consolidation.

3. Look carefully at the nature of the shadowing. In consolidation the alveolar spaces become filled with fluid making them appear white, whereas the airways retain air making them appear black. If you look closely at an area of consolidation you can often make out the small airways as black against a white background – the so-called 'air bronchogram'.

4. Look at the distribution of the shadowing. Fluid sinks, so consolidation gets denser as one moves down the lung. The shadowing in consolidation will often be denser and more clearly demarcated at its lower border.

If a patient is admitted with pneumonia it is not necessary to repeat the chest X-ray before discharge if they make a satisfactory recovery. For patients who fail to recover, further X-rays are necessary to look for possible complications such as the development of an empyema or pulmonary abscess. For patients ill enough to warrant admission to intensive care, early follow-up X-rays are warranted to ensure that their condition is not progressing.

All patients should be reviewed after 6 weeks. If they have persistent symptoms or signs or are at risk of malignancy (smokers and those over 50 years of age) a follow-up X-ray should be arranged to ensure complete resolution. If there is persistent consolidation at this stage, further investigations should be arranged to exclude malignancy.

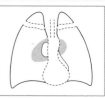

**4.4 *Pneumocystis carinii (jiroveci)*
pneumonia (PCP)**

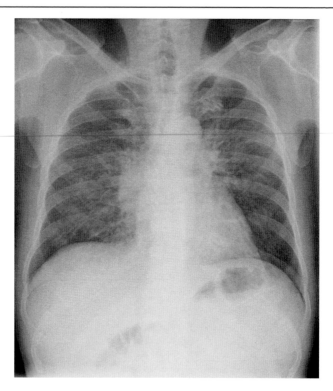

This patient is on long-term immunosuppression following renal transplant. He presented with a week-long history of a dry cough and increasing breathlessness. Following bronchoscopy and lavage he was diagnosed with *Pneumocystis* pneumonia, an organism recognized to cause pneumonia in immune compromise from many causes.

The film shows vague white shadowing around the hilum. There is also enlargement of the right hilum from lymphadenopathy.

Pneumocystis carinii pneumonia (PCP) can be difficult to diagnose on a chest X-ray and in 10% of patients with PCP the chest X-ray is normal. It is something to suspect if a patient presents with shortness of breath and hypoxia which are out of proportion to a relatively normal looking chest X-ray.

If you suspect that the chest X-ray shadowing may be due to PCP then look for the following features:

1. Look at lung volumes. Very early PCP may be suspected when both lungs show reduced volume. Look for an old chest X-ray. If there is one, compare the lung volumes to a chest X-ray taken when the patient was well.

2. Look at the area around the hilum. In PCP there is often white shadowing in this region. This can be very vague. You can best appreciate it by looking at the blood vessels as they come away from the hila. In PCP the blood vessels will appear less well defined than normal.

3. Look for peribronchial cuffing. This is best seen in airways that are seen 'end-on' and is due to fluid seen as increased whiteness within the walls of the airways. This gives the wall of the airway a thickened or fuzzy appearance, with a central hole, rather like a well-sucked 'Polo' mint.

4. Look for large areas of whiteness extending throughout the lung fields. These may develop as the disease progresses and represent large areas of consolidation. Typically, in PCP the whiteness does not extend to the apices or affect the costophrenic angles.

4.5 Pleural effusion

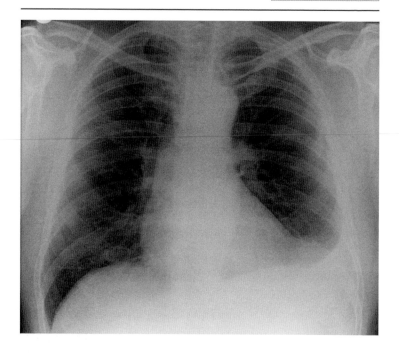

This pair of films shows the varied appearances of pleural effusions. The first film shows a small left effusion filling the costophrenic angle. It has a curved upper margin.

The second film shows a much larger right pleural effusion. The fluid now encases the lung and the increased whiteness can be seen around the apex of the lung. Compare this almost totally white lung with the appearance following a pneumonectomy. In the case of a large pleural effusion, the mediastinum may be pushed away from the midline by the large volume of fluid.

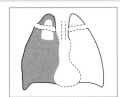

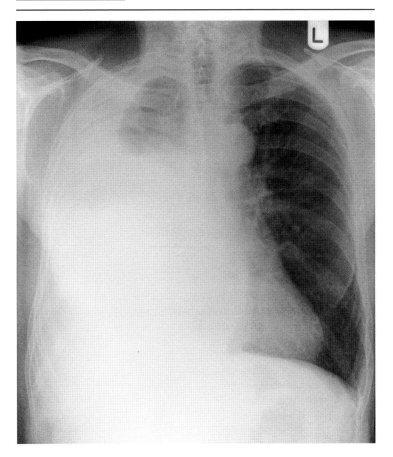

If you see an area of whiteness at the base of a lung then the possible causes are a pleural effusion, a raised hemidiaphragm and an area of consolidation or collapse. You need to determine which of these it is.

1. Look closely at the texture of the whiteness. Consolidation usually causes more heterogeneous shadowing, typically with the presence of an air bronchogram. Look carefully for an air bronchogram (p. 60) since its presence will point to consolidation rather than a pleural effusion.

2. Look at the shape of the upper border of the shadowing. Fluid will have a meniscus so the upper outer border of an effusion will be concave.

3. To differentiate an effusion from a raised hemidiaphragm look again at the shape of the upper border. The upper border of an effusion will peak much more laterally than you would expect the diaphragm to do. This is a matter of looking at lots of X-rays.

4. Look for mediastinal shift. It can be difficult to differentiate an effusion from lung collapse. Collapse usually causes mediastinal shift towards the white lung field so the absence of shift suggests the presence of an effusion. Remember, however, that collapse can accompany an effusion so that, although the absence of shift implies an effusion, its presence does not exclude it.

5. A lateral view is often helpful since the meniscus on a lateral can be much more obvious. Look for the presence of a meniscus which, often on the lateral, is seen to extend up into one of the fissures.

6. If you diagnose an effusion look on the X-ray for possible causes. Check the size of the heart (a large heart points to heart failure) and look at the hilum for possible enlargement. Look at the visible parts of the lung fields for obvious masses and check the bones for signs of metastasis. Look very carefully at the apices of the lungs for tumours and TB.

7. To confirm the presence of pleural fluid request an ultrasound of the chest. This is particularly important if you plan to aspirate the effusion or put in a chest drain.

Some causes of a pleural effusion

Transudate <30 g/l of protein

Heart failure, e.g. congestive cardiac failure, pericardial effusion
Liver failure, e.g. cirrhosis
Protein loss, e.g. nephrotic syndrome, protein losing enteritis
Reduced protein intake, e.g. malnutrition
Iatrogenic, e.g. peritoneal dialysis

Exudate >30 g/l of protein

Infection, e.g. pneumonia, tuberculosis
Infarction
Malignancy, e.g. bronchial carcinoma, mesothelioma, metastasis
Collagen vascular disease, e.g. rheumatoid arthritis, SLE
Abdominal disease, e.g. pancreatitis, subphrenic abscess
Trauma/surgery

4.6 Asbestos plaques

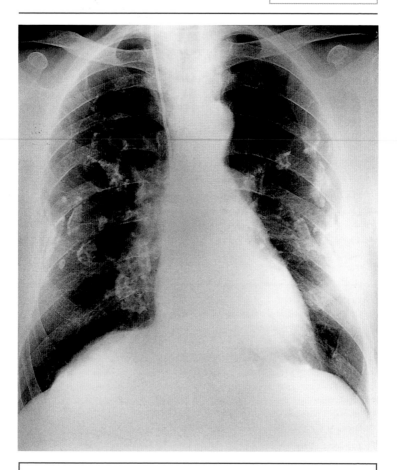

This is the chest film of a 63-year-old man admitted following a gastrointestinal haemorrhage (hence the central venous pressure line) who had been exposed to asbestos whilst working in a naval dockyard. You can see multiple calcified pleural plaques on the inner chest wall.

Pleural plaques represent areas of pleural thickening caused by exposure to asbestos fibres. They may be predominantly soft tissue with small amounts of calcium or be heavily calcified. Isolated pleural thickening is a cause of a localized area of white lung and can be difficult to separate from lung shadows. If you suspect pleural plaques then:

1. Look throughout the lung fields of both lungs. Pleural thickening is easy to identify at the periphery where it appears as a thickened line around the edge of the lung. If you can identify pleural thickening here it makes it more likely that the other areas of whiteness are plaques superimposed over the lung field.

2. Carefully look at the position of the whiteness and compare it to what you know of the anatomy of the lung. If the whiteness follows intrapulmonary structures, for example a lobe of the lung, then it may be originating from the lung itself. If it crosses such structures then it is probably pleural.

3. Compare the distribution of the whiteness to the line of the anterior portion of the ribs. Asbestos plaques are very commonly found running along the line of the anterior portion of the ribs.

4. Look at the distribution of the patches. Pleural plaques are most prevalent in the mid zones and axillary region of the mid chest. They tend to spare the upper zones and costophrenic angles. Look carefully at both lung fields. Pleural plaques are usually bilateral and you should be wary of making this diagnosis if they are present in only one pleural cavity.

5. Look at the diaphragm. Pleural plaques along the diaphragm are often calcified. If you see streaks of dense white material (calcium) running along the diaphragm it implies that pleural plaques are present.

6. Look at the nature of the whiteness. Pleural plaques are patchy in nature as opposed to a pleural effusion which is more uniform. Plaques are sometimes said to have a map-like appearance due to areas of patchy calcification within them. Look at their edge. This should be well defined as opposed to 'companion shadows' that have poorly defined margins.

7. Look at old X-rays. Pleural plaques are slow growing and are probably visible on previous X-rays.

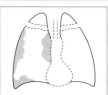

4.7 Mesothelioma

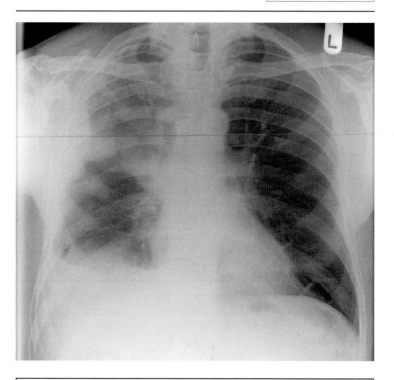

This is the chest X-ray of a 68-year-old man with a history of asbestos exposure. He presented with right lateral chest wall pains. The film demonstrates lobulated pleural thickening around the upper, mid and basal right lung, with further pleural thickening evident next to the right side of the mediastinum. CT of a mesothelioma in a different patient is shown on page 71.

Mesothelioma is a malignant tumour of the pleura. The shadowing it causes will have the characteristics of pleural shadowing and some of the characteristics of malignant shadows. If you suspect the whiteness to be mesothelioma then:

1. Look carefully at the spread of the whiteness and determine whether it follows lung boundaries. If it does not, then the whiteness may be pleural in origin.

2. Look at the margins of the whiteness. If they are lobulated in nature, then this suggests malignancy.

3. Look at the upper edge of the whiteness. The main differential is a pleural effusion. A pleural effusion would be unlikely if the upper edge was lobulated and no meniscus was visible.

4. Compare the volume of the affected side. Loss of volume on the affected side may increase your suspicions of a mesothelioma.

Pleural tumours

Mesothelioma
Primary pleural adenocarcinoma
Pleural sarcoma
Pleural fibromas
Neurofibromas arising paravertebrally or in relation to an intercostal nerve
Secondaries

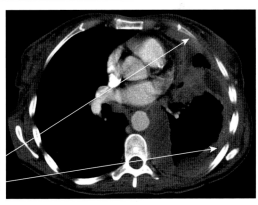

Extensive pleural thickening encasing the lung, and tracking into the fissures

4.8 Pleural disease on a CT scan

The pleura should not really be visible on a CT scan, since they are so thin. If you see an increased grey area on the inner surface of the chest wall, then suspect that the patient may have pleural disease. Pleural abnormalities are best seen on a spiral CT.

Remember, the pleura is in two layers with a potential space in between. Pleural thickening can affect the visceral (next to the lung) or the parietal (next to the chest wall) pleura. The double layers of pleura run into and out of the fissures of the lung.

If you see increased density around the inner chest wall:

1. Look at the colour of the pleural density on the soft tissue window.

   a. Is it grey? The commonest pleural abnormality is pleural fluid. This will appear darker than the muscles of the chest wall. If the pleural density is the same as the chest wall, it is more likely to be pleural thickening.

   b. Is it white? This is more likely to be pleural calcification. Pleural plaques often contain very bright white areas where they have calcified.

2. Are the margins of the pleural density smooth or lobulated?

   a. Does it have smooth margins? This may be pleural fluid or pleural thickening. Multiple discrete lesions that are short but quite deep are probably pleural plaques.

   b. Does it have lobulated margins? This is more likely to be a malignancy.

3. Is the pleural density very extensive or patchy?

   a. Benign pleural thickening and malignant pleural diseases, especially mesothelioma (p. 71), will give a much more diffuse thickening extending over a much greater area of pleura.

   b. Pleural plaques are smaller (usually 1–4 cm in length) and well defined. As both pleural plaques and mesothelioma can occur following asbestos exposure, the two may be found together.

4. Look at the position. A small pleural effusion will usually lie against the posterior chest wall as the patient is lying flat for the CT. A larger pleural effusion will surround the lung and compress it, causing some of the outer regions of the lung to become solid. This fluid can track into the fissures.

5. Look at the 'normal' pleura. With an empyema, if a contrast-enhanced scan has been performed, as well as the grey fluid the pleura may 'enhance' and appear whiter than normal.

Simple pleural effusion

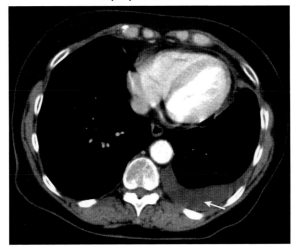

Benign pleural plaques

Pleural plaques, discrete, partly soft tissue, partly calcified

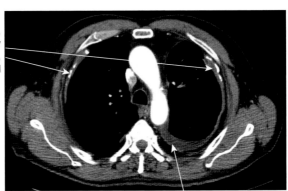

Benign type pleural effusion

4.9 Lung nodule

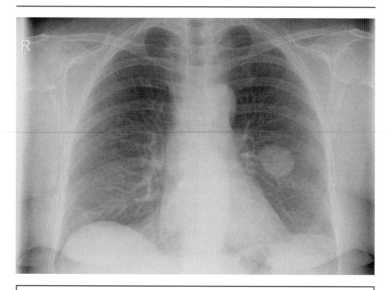

There is a 3 cm round nodule in the left mid zone. This would need to be investigated as it may represent a small tumour. If bronchoscopy does not provide the answer, the nodule could be biopsied percutaneously under CT guidance.

The term 'lung nodule' is used to describe a discrete area of whiteness situated within a lung field. It is less than 3 cm in diameter. It is not necessarily strictly circular. The main worry is that it may represent a carcinoma. Other possibilities are a localized area of consolidation, an abscess or a pleural abnormality. Go through the following steps in assessing the abnormality:

1. Look at the edge of the lesion. A spiculated, irregular or lobulated edge is suggestive of malignancy.

2. Look for areas of calcification. These would be dense white (the same density as bone) and be obviously much denser than the rest of the lesion. Calcification is rare in a malignant lesion and would point you to an alternative diagnosis.

3. Look at the nature of the whiteness. If the lesion is cavitating the centre may be darker than the circumference. If looking at an X-ray film, stand back from the X-ray since a cavity is often easier to see from a distance.

4. Look for an air bronchogram. This is a sign of consolidation and so would be a most unusual finding if the lesion was a tumour.

5. Look for other coin nodules. The presence of more than one strongly suggests metastatic disease.

6. Look for abnormalities peripheral to the lesion. A tumour may cause problems distal to it such as infection causing consolidation or an area of collapse.

7. Look carefully at the rest of the X-ray. Malignant tumours may be associated with mediastinal lymphadenopathy or bone metastasis.

8. Look at old films if available. Tumours grow, and so if the lesion was present on an earlier film compare its size. Some tumours grow slowly, but it is safe to say that if the lesion has not changed over a period of two years or greater it is unlikely to be malignant.

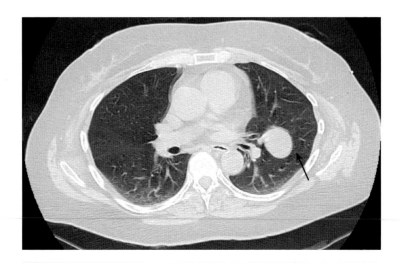

The arrow marks the location of the left oblique fissure. The coin lesion seen on the plain film lies on the oblique fissure and in front of it. The remainder of the CT scan showed no evidence of metastatic disease and no hilar or mediastinal lymph nodes were involved. The patient was referred for a PET scan and subsequently underwent a left upper lobectomy.

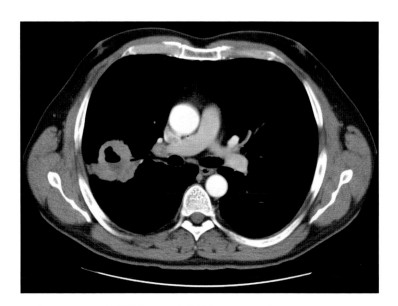

Here we can see a nodule with a black centre indicating that it has cavitated.
This was proven to be a squamous cell carcinoma.

Causes of solitary pulmonary nodules

Benign tumour, e.g. hamartoma
Malignant tumour, e.g. bronchial carcinoma, single secondary
Infection, e.g. pneumonia, abscess, tuberculosis, hydatid cyst
Infarction
Rheumatoid nodule

4.10 Cavitating lung lesion

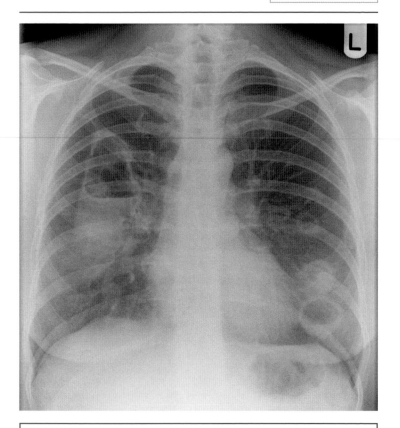

These two films both demonstrate cavitating lung lesions. In the first study there are bilateral thin-walled cavities, some with air–fluid levels. This was due to Wegener's granulomatosis.

The second film shows a single cavitating mass lesion in the left mid zone. This has a much thicker wall. This lesion was found to be due to a cavitating tumour. The thickness of the wall makes this a more likely diagnosis.

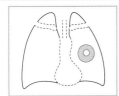

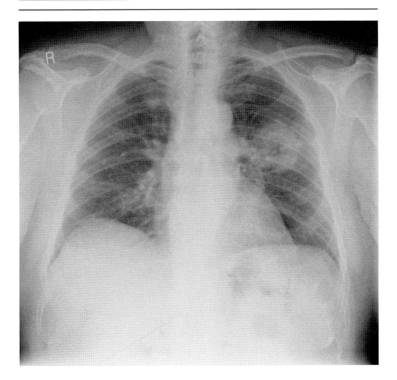

Some coin lesions may cavitate, and if you have identified a coin lesion, it is important to look for the features of cavitation. Therefore:

1. Look at the centre of the lesion and compare it to the periphery. If the centre is darker this points to cavitation.

2. Look for a fluid level. Look for a horizontal line within the lesion. There will be whiteness (fluid) below the line with an area of black (air) above. Fluid levels are common in cavities and their presence should suggest one.

3. Look at the lateral film. Cavities and fluid levels are often easier to see on a lateral, especially when they are posterior or inferior in position.

4. Look at old films. If the lesion is longstanding, it may be possible to see the cavity developing.

If you diagnose a cavitating lesion:

1. Look at the wall of the cavity. It is often said that cavity walls are thicker (>5 mm) when the lesion is a neoplasm as opposed to an abscess. This rule does not always hold, but the thicker the wall the more likely it is that the lesion is neoplastic.

2. Look carefully at the inside of the cavity. If there appears to be a white ball within it, this is characteristic of an aspergilloma.

Causes of cavitating lung lesions

Abscess
Neoplasm
Cavitation around a pneumonia
Infarct
Wegener's disease
Rheumatoid nodules (rare)

4.11 Left ventricular failure (LVF)

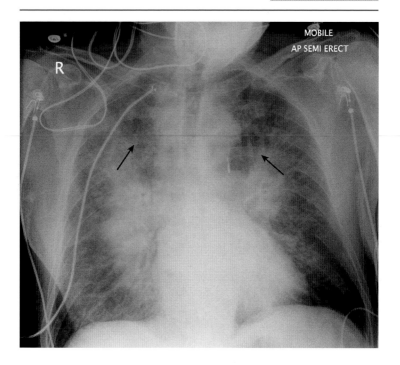

This patient presented with an acute cardiac event. At present the pleural spaces are clear but it is common in pulmonary oedema to develop pleural effusions. These are often larger on the right than on the left. Pulmonary upper zone blood vessels are also often dilated, as is shown in this film (arrows). This patient's film clearly shows 'bat's wing' hilar shadows characteristic of pulmonary oedema. The magnified image of the right lower zone (opposite) shows the horizontal septal lines more clearly (arrowed).

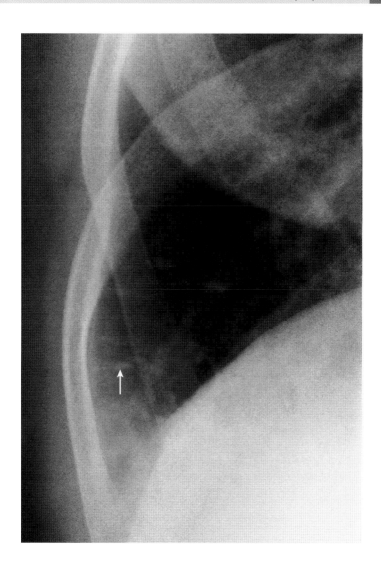

If you suspect heart failure as a cause of a generalized, or localized, area of shadowing then:

1. Look at the size of the heart. The presence of left ventricular dilatation is strongly suggestive of heart failure. In a PA film the maximum diameter of the heart should be less than half that of the maximum diameter of the thorax (the cardiothoracic ratio). If it exceeds this, then there is a cardiac abnormality, such as left ventricular enlargement, and this suggests that the associated shadowing is due to LVF (see Chapter 7 for other causes of an enlarged cardiac shadow). You cannot comment on the size of the heart on an AP portable film since the heart is anterior and will appear magnified. Note also that in acute onset LVF you may not get cardiac enlargement.

2. Look for Kerley B lines. These are caused by oedema of the interlobular septa. They are horizontal, non-branching, white lines best seen at the periphery of the lung just above the costophrenic angle.

3. Compare the size of the upper lobe and lower lobe blood vessels. Take an upper lobe and a lower lobe blood vessel at similar distances from the hilum and compare their widths. The upper should be narrower than the lower. If they are the same size or the upper is wider there is upper lobe blood diversion – the first sign of heart failure. Note that this only applies to an erect film. Upper lobe blood diversion is normal on a supine film and not suggestive of heart failure – a common mistake.

Upper lobe blood diversion is due to lower zone arteriolar vasoconstriction secondary to alveolar hypoxia.

Severe heart failure

Severe pulmonary oedema gives confluent alveolar shadowing which spreads out from the hilum giving a 'bat's wing' appearance. If this is the cause of generalized shadowing then upper lobe blood diversion and Kerley B lines may be present. Look also at the hilum. In pulmonary oedema it may appear distended and the vessels close to the hilum may be blurred.

Severe heart failure vs non-cardiogenic pulmonary oedema

It can be difficult to distinguish non-cardiogenic pulmonary oedema (acute respiratory distress syndrome) from LVF. In non-cardiogenic pulmonary oedema the heart size is likely to be normal (though see 1 above) and there will not necessarily be sparing of the peripheries. (See also Chapter 4.12.)

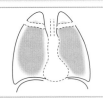

4.12 Acute respiratory distress syndrome

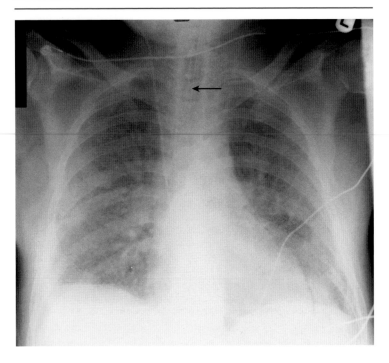

This 36-year-old man presented with severe upper abdominal pain and was diagnosed as having pancreatitis. Whilst in hospital he became acutely short of breath and required intubation and ventilation. Note the ET tube (arrowed). A chest X-ray was taken which suggested that he had developed the complication of acute respiratory distress syndrome (ARDS). Note that the X-ray shows multiple bilateral white shadows but does not have any signs of left ventricular failure. Unfortunately this man died after 3 weeks of mechanical ventilation on the intensive care unit.

Acute respiratory distress syndrome (ARDS) is defined as respiratory failure in association with a chest X-ray that shows confluent alveolar opacification (whitening) of the lungs that looks like pulmonary oedema.

The other (and far more common) cause of pulmonary oedema is left ventricular failure which is also a cause of respiratory failure. Therefore, if you see a chest X-ray that has bilateral white shadows in the lungs and you suspect ARDS look for the following clues:

1. Look at the distribution of the shadowing. In ARDS it should be present in both lungs – that is part of the definition. Look also at the nature of the shadowing. It is usually fairly ill-defined which means it is difficult to see a clear edge. It may also have the features of consolidation which means that you may be able to see an air bronchogram within it (p. 60).

2. To distinguish ARDS from left ventricular failure:

a. Look at the heart size. In left ventricular failure you would expect the heart to be big. In ARDS it may be normal size.

b. Look again at the distribution of the shadowing. In left ventricular failure it tends to be more central whereas in ARDS it is more peripheral.

c. Look for Kerley B lines (see p. 84). Although these do occur in ARDS they are far more common in left ventricular failure.

d. Look for the presence of a pleural effusion. These may be small so look carefully at the edge of the diaphragm for loss of the normal costophrenic angle. Pleural effusions can occur in ARDS but they are much more common in left ventricular failure.

e. Look at old films. A large heart and pleural effusion may have shown on earlier films and may point to left ventricular failure as a more likely diagnosis.

If you are certain that the chest X-ray suggests a diagnosis of ARDS then look for clues as to the cause. There are many causes of ARDS (see Box on p. 89) and most can only be picked up by history and examination. However, an asymmetrical distribution of the shadowing, i.e. significantly more shadowing in one lung than the other, may point to lung injury as a cause. Chest X-rays taken just before the development of ARDS may show an obvious pneumonia.

Some causes of ARDS

ARDS is caused by any insult to either the alveolar or endothelial cells that results in a loss of integrity of the junction between those cells allowing fluid to leak into the alveoli. Causes include:

Aspiration including toxic gas inhalation	Drugs, including drugs of abuse
Lung trauma	Drowning
Pneumonia	Fat embolism after trauma
Radiation	Hypersensitivity reactions
Sepsis	Transfusion reactions

Complications of ARDS

A patient with ARDS should have their chest X-ray repeated daily. Look for signs of disease progression or resolution. Look also for the development of a pneumothorax or lung cysts due to barotraumas caused by the use of positive pressure ventilation in the treatment of ARDS.

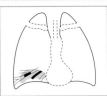

4.13 Bronchiectasis

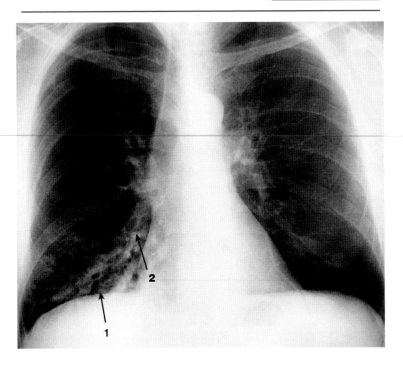

This film shows a localized area of bronchiectasis in the right lower lobe which has resulted from earlier pertussis infection. In the lower lobe you can see a cluster of typical ring shadows giving a 'bunches of grapes' appearance (1) together with bronchial wall thickening seen side-on, which gives two thick parallel lines, known as tramline shadows (2).

Bronchiectasis can be difficult to diagnose on a plain chest X-ray. If you suspect it as a cause of increased shadowing then look for the following features:

1. *Ring shadows.* These look like rings and are any size up to 1 cm in diameter. They can be single but usually occur in groups giving a 'bunches of grapes' appearance. Ring shadows represent diseased bronchi seen end on.

2. *Tramline shadows.* Look for these towards the periphery of the lung. They consist of two thick white parallel lines separated by black. It is common to get parallel lines close to the hilum in the normal chest X-ray but these lines are hairline in nature. True tramline shadowing is thicker and is not necessarily close to the hilum. Tramline shadows are diseased bronchi seen side on.

3. *Tubular shadows.* These are solid thick white shadows up to 8 mm wide. They represent bronchi filled with secretions seen side on. They are not common but their presence suggests bronchiectasis.

4. *Glove finger shadows.* These represent a group of tubular shadows seen head on and look like the fingers of a glove – hence the name!

The presence of any of these features suggests the possibility of bronchiectasis. A normal chest X-ray does not, however, exclude the diagnosis and CT scanning is the most sensitive diagnostic test available.

The HRCT scan and bronchiectasis

Although bronchiectasis can be diagnosed on a plain chest X-ray, in half the patients the X-ray is normal. Therefore, if you suspect bronchiectasis and the chest X-ray is normal, you will need to undertake a high-resolution CT (HRCT) scan. An HRCT scan may also give you clues as to the cause of the bronchiectasis and will give you a much more accurate picture of the extent of disease.

To diagnose bronchiectasis on HRCT scanning you need to identify areas in which the bronchi are dilated. There are a number of ways of doing this. Look at the lung windows:

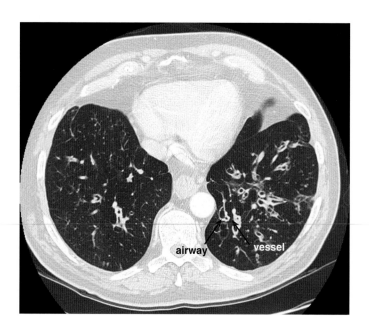

1. Look in the periphery of the lung, where the airways are round. Compare the airway diameter here to that of the neighbouring blood vessels. If the diameter of the airway is larger than that of the neighbouring blood vessel, then it is dilated. The airway is usually patent so will have a black hole in the middle whereas the blood vessel is solid white.

2. Look in the middle third of the lung fields. The airways here can be seen along their long axis, and the airway walls should normally taper over 2 cm. If there is no tapering, this is a sign of more proximal airway dilatation.

3. Look for areas of mucus plugging. These are airways in which the lumen has been blocked by mucus. The normal airway has the appearance of a white ring (the airway wall) surrounding a black hole (the air within the airway). When the airway is plugged it has

a solid appearance – the plug, being mucus, may have a lower density (be darker) than the airway wall when you look at the mediastinal windows. Occasionally it is not clear whether these structures are impacted airways or blood vessels since both may appear white.

4. Look at the lung parenchyma around the airways, since changes in the lung occur around bronchiectatic airways. These changes include:

- areas of collapse, known as atelectasis
- areas of very small airway plugging, known as 'tree in bud'
- larger patches of consolidation.

The HRCT scan may also give some clues as to the cause of the bronchiectasis. The radiologist will look at the distribution of the changes to give an indication of the possible aetiology. For example:

- If it is localized to one lobe or one segment of lung it could be due to an obstructive lesion which would require further investigation by a contiguous CT scan and a bronchoscopy to find the cause.
- Proximal bronchiectasis is often seen in allergic bronchopulmonary aspergillosis (ABPA).
- Cystic fibrosis causes widespread bronchiectasis often more marked in the upper zones, with some sparing of the lung bases.

Finally, when looking at the scan, you should note the extent of the disease. Mild bronchiectasis is a relatively common finding on HRCT and may not necessarily be the cause of the patient's symptoms. Interpret the scan in the context of the clinical history and make sure that you discuss the images with a radiologist.

Some causes of bronchiectasis

Structural, e.g. obstruction (carcinoma, foreign body)
Infection, e.g. childhood pertussis or measles, tuberculosis, pneumonia
Immune, e.g. hypogammaglobulinaemia, allergic bronchopulmonary aspergillosis
Congenital, e.g. cystic fibrosis
Idiopathic

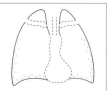

4.14 Fibrosis

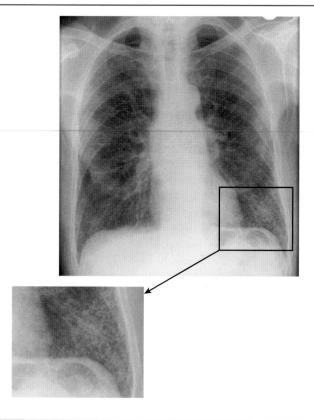

This patient has pulmonary fibrosis and as there is no known predisposing cause it is termed cryptogenic fibrosing alveolitis (CFA). The film demonstrates a fine meshwork pattern over the lungs which is worse in the periphery of the lungs, especially at the lung bases. In very severely affected areas a denser meshwork produces a 'honeycomb' appearance.

Fibrosis is one of the rarer causes of white lung and you need to differentiate it from consolidation or oedema which is far more common. If you suspect fibrosis:

1. Look at old X-rays if possible. Fibrosis is a fairly chronic process so if present a while ago it is more likely to be fibrosis than consolidation or oedema.

2. Look at the distribution of the shadowing. This may help differentiate fibrosis from oedema since the latter is more likely to be bilateral, basal and peripheral. Shadowing that is bilateral and basal could be either oedema or fibrosis. Shadowing that is mid zone or apical is more likely to be fibrosis.

3. Look at the size of the lungs. Fibrosis may cause shrinkage of the lungs which will not be caused by consolidation or oedema. The presence of small lungs points strongly to fibrosis.

4. Look at the shape of the mediastinum. Since fibrosis causes shrinkage of the lungs it will pull the mediastinum and distort the outline.

5. Look at the nature of the shadowing. Pulmonary fibrosis gives reticular-nodular shadowing which simply means a meshwork of lines that combine to form nodules and ring shadows of about 5 mm in diameter. Sometimes the meshwork is very fine giving a ground-glass appearance, said to look like a thin veil over the lung. Later it gives a more coarse appearance and is said to look like a honeycomb. Compare this appearance to that of pulmonary oedema (p. 82) or consolidation (p. 58) and you will see that it is quite distinctive, although in fact it is the other features of fibrosis outlined above that are often the most useful in making the diagnosis.

6. Look at the heart border and diaphragm. Both of these may appear blurred if fibrosis is present.

7. Look at the vascular markings. These become less distinct in areas of fibrosis. This is due to the development of numerous small areas of lung collapse.

The HRCT scan and pulmonary fibrosis

HRCT is the established test for patients with pulmonary fibrosis. It is a more sensitive and specific test than a plain chest X-ray. If there is clinical suspicion and the patient has a normal X-ray you should still order a HRCT. The scan will demonstrate the distribution and character of fibrosis. This can give valuable clues as to its aetiology and is a sensitive way to follow disease progression.

You will be ordering the scan to give you details of any lung paren-chymal changes. Therefore you will need to order a high-resolution scan so that you can see the fine detail of the lung architecture.

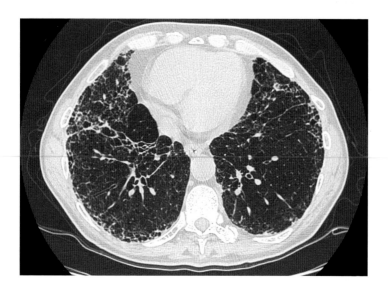

On the CT image the small black holes around the lung edges are the honey-comb pattern. Another feature seen on CT is that the fibrosis causes changes in other structures in the lung, for instance the airways are pulled apart and the usual smooth curve of the fissure is lost.

Confirming fibrosis

1. Look at the surface of the pleura. One of the first changes is the development of small irregular lumps on the pulmonary surface of the pleura.

2. Look for septal lines. These are thin white lines, 1–2 cm in length, that are perpendicular to the pleura.

3. Look at the bronchi. In pulmonary fibrosis there is a lot of inflammation in the lung around the airway, and this can pull the airway walls apart. Unlike in bronchiectasis, the walls do not appear thickened. This is known as traction airway change.

4. Look for very small lung nodules that can occur. They may be well defined or be slightly hazy in their appearance. In sarcoidosis nodules may coalesce in the lung to form masses and they may also be seen along the fissures, known as 'beading'.

5. The meshwork of lines in the lung periphery may give rise to a 'honeycomb' appearance. This occurs late on in the fibrotic process and consists of areas of black air surrounded by a thicker white border.

6. Look for a ground glass density in the lung. This has a very specific appearance. There is abnormal increased whiteness in the lung. Look at the blood vessels – with ground glass shadowing the blood vessels must still be visible. If they cannot be seen then that area of lung is said to be consolidated (another cause of increased whiteness in the lung). Ground glass density tends to be unevenly distributed through the lung – it may affect particular zones of the lung or occur in smaller discrete areas. Ground glass density may represent very fine fibrotic change which is below the resolution of the scanner to demonstrate more clearly or conversely be due to transient abnormalities such as infection or fluid within the lung. If seen in isolation it is difficult to be certain of its significance, but if seen with the other features described above it is consistent with an interstitial fibrosis.

Determining aetiology

A radiologist may be able to determine the aetiology of pulmonary fibrosis by careful examination of the HRCT images. They will look for a number of clues, for example:

1. The distribution of the fibrotic changes.

    a. Idiopathic pulmonary fibrosis, fibrosis secondary to connective tissue disease, and asbestosis are characterized by their patchy distribution and by the presence of subpleural, predominantly basal, fibrotic changes.

    b. Sarcoidosis causes changes predominantly in the mid zones and around the hila.

2. The appearance of the interlobular septa. In lymphangitis carcino-matosis there is irregular thickening of the interlobular septa. Some nodular deposits can also be seen on the pleura, but the distribution is not usually the same as that of sarcoidosis.

3. The appearance of the pleura. In asbestos lung diseases the pulmo-nary fibrosis is often accompanied by changes to the pleura, notably pleural thickening and calcified pleural plaques.

4. Mediastinal changes.

    a. In sarcoidosis the scan may confirm bilateral hilar lymphadenopathy.

    b. Fibrosing alveolitis is often accompanied by lymph node enlarge-ment in the mediastinum.

The HRCT scan can accurately determine the aetiology of interstitial lung disease. However, this accuracy is highly dependent on the skill of the interpreter and so it is vital that these scans are assessed by experienced radiologists.

Causes of fibrosis

Cryptogenic
External/occupational, e.g. extrinsic allergic alveolitis, asbestosis
Infection, e.g. tuberculosis, psittacosis, aspiration pneumonia
Collagen vascular, e.g. rheumatoid arthritis, systemic lupus erythematosus (SLE)
Sarcoid
Iatrogenic, e.g. amiodarone, busulfan, radiotherapy

4.15 Chickenpox pneumonia

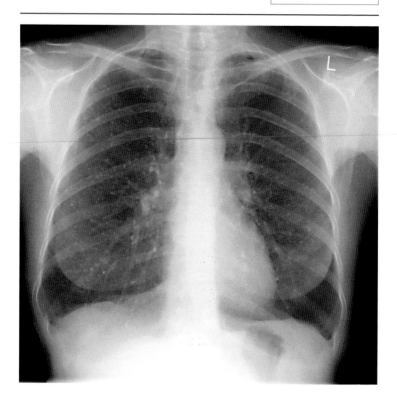

This film of a woman admitted with an acute abdomen shows the typical appearance of old chickenpox pneumonia. You can see numerous bilateral calcified intrapulmonary nodules.

Chickenpox pneumonia in adulthood can cause the development of numerous calcified nodules. To determine whether this is a likely diagnosis:

1. Look at the distribution of the nodules. In chickenpox pneumonia they tend to be in the lower and mid zones.

2. Look at the density of the nodules. They are calcified and so should be very white in appearance.

3. Look at their size. They are usually less than 3 mm in diameter.

Causes of numerous calcified nodules

Infection, e.g. TB, histoplasmosis, chickenpox
Inhalation, e.g. silicosis
Chronic renal failure
Lymphoma following radiotherapy
Chronic pulmonary venous hypertension in mitral stenosis

4.16 Miliary shadowing

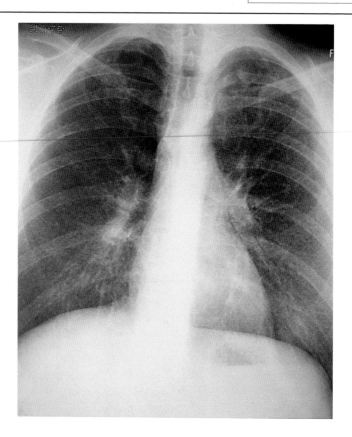

This is the chest film of a 32-year-old man with immunodeficiency. It shows the typical miliary shadowing characteristic of tuberculosis (TB). There is also soft shadowing in the left apex consistent with TB.

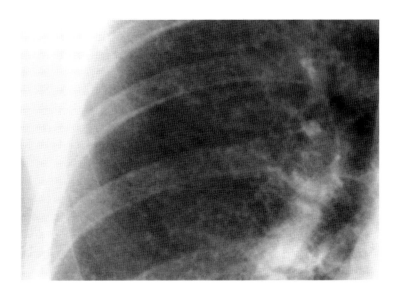

The lungs have a spotted appearance. This may be due to miliary shadowing. The normal lung can sometimes have a mottled appearance. This can be especially so in obese patients. To distinguish between miliary shadowing and normal lung:

1. Look at the distribution of the shadowing. Look carefully at the periphery. If the shadowing is present in the periphery it is far more likely to be pathological. Sometimes normal vasculature can mimic interstitial shadowing but this usually occurs only towards the centre of the lung fields.

2. Move close to the X-ray and carefully examine the shadowing. With miliary shadowing the opacities should be discrete. Noise from overlying soft tissue can appear more fuzzy.

3. Compare a few of the opacities with one another. If the shadowing is miliary they should be of a similar density and size.

If you feel the shadowing is miliary then look for clues as to its cause. Likely possibilities are miliary TB, sarcoid or malignant miliary metastasis:

1. Look again at the distribution. With miliary TB the opacities are most profuse in the upper zone, with sarcoid they are most profuse

in the perihilar and mid zones, and with miliary metastases there may be more opacities in the lower zone.

2. Look at the density. High density, very white shadows are likely to be dust related industrial disease or calcified TB. Less dense changes could be multiple secondaries, sarcoid or any of the other causes of miliary mottling.

3. Look at the rest of the X-ray for signs of other disease processes. Look at the hilum. Unilateral hilar enlargement suggests TB and bilateral hilar enlargement sarcoidosis. Look at the upper part of the mediastinum for thyroid enlargement which could suggest secondaries from a thyroid carcinoma. Look at the apices for subtle cavitating lesions suggestive of TB. Note, however, that the presence of apical shadowing, although suggestive of TB, is in fact very rare in patients with miliary spread.

CHAPTER 5

The black lung field

5.1 Chronic obstructive pulmonary
disease 106

5.2 Pneumothorax 110

5.3 Tension pneumothorax 112

5.4 Pulmonary embolus 114

5.5 Mastectomy 119

5.1 Chronic obstructive pulmonary disease (COPD)

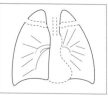

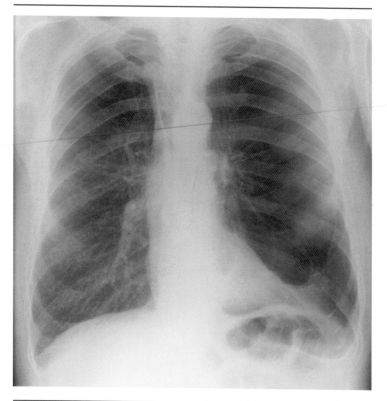

This is the chest film of a patient with chronic obstructive pulmonary disease. The lungs look larger in volume than normal. The diaphragms are rather flattened. The right upper zone and many areas of the left lung are abnormally black. In these areas the blood vessels are difficult to see or are very thinned. This is because these regions of lung have developed emphysema.

The CT section shows how the lung contains black holes (1) and thin thready blood vessels (2).

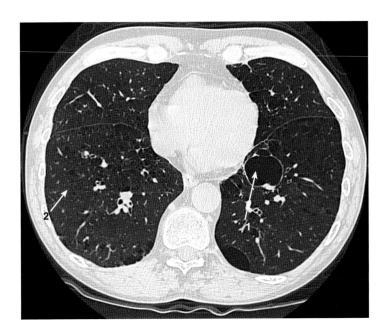

When trying to decide the cause of *bilateral* black lungs you need to:

1. Check the penetration. Look at the vertebral bodies behind the heart. Remember that in a good quality X-ray the vertebral bodies become harder to see behind the heart shadow. If they are too clearly seen the film is over penetrated making the lungs appear black.

If you are satisfied with the technical quality of the film then the most likely cause is COPD. COPD is associated with large lungs due to air trapping and the development of bullae. You therefore need to:

1. Look at the shape of the diaphragm. In COPD the diaphragms are flat or even scallop shaped instead of concave upwards. This is a more reliable sign of hyperexpansion than rib counting.

2. Count the number of ribs you see anteriorly. If the lungs are enlarged you should be able to count more than seven. Be careful, however, because you can sometimes count more than seven ribs in normal patients if they are tall and slim.

3. Look at the shape of the heart. The enlarged thorax of COPD appears on the X-ray to elongate and narrow the heart, elevating the lower border. The heart, instead of sitting on the diaphragm, often appears to 'swing in the wind'. It will also appear small unless there is also an element of cardiac failure in which case it will be normal in size or large.

4. Look for bullae. These are densely black areas of lung, usually round, surrounded by fine curvilinear shadows. Bullae distort the surrounding vasculature so to help find them look out for areas of distortion of vascular markings.

5. Look at the distribution of lung markings. The black lungs of COPD are due to reduced size of blood vessels. The lung markings are reduced bilaterally and fan out in straight lines from the hilum, starting off chunky but stopping two-thirds of the way out – peripheral pruning.

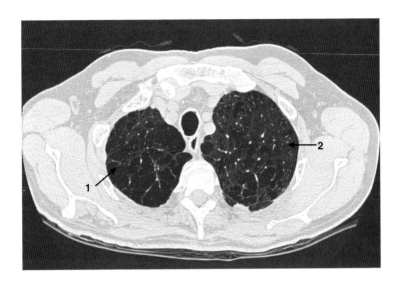

Cigarette smoking causes damage to the parenchyma of the lung. Cigarette smoke in a room tends to float upwards, and similarly smoking related lung damage tends to occur in the upper lungs. This image shows how the normal smooth lung texture has been destroyed with the formation of air cysts (bullae – 1) and small black holes in the lung (centrilobular emphysema – 2). The blood vessels through these areas can also become very narrowed, as the body will not perfuse areas of the lung where gas exchange is significantly impaired.

5.2 Pneumothorax

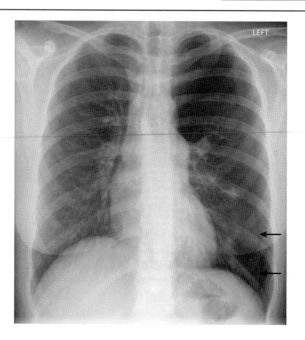

This patient has a left-sided pneumothorax with partial collapse of the left lung. The outer left lung field is black. You can see the lung edge (arrowed).

When you see a *unilateral* black lung you need to:

1. Check the technical quality of the film. A rotated film may make one side less dense than the other.

2. Determine which side is abnormal. This is usually easy since the side with reduced lung markings will be the abnormal side.

You must now decide the cause of the blackness. Lung markings are made up of bronchi and blood vessels and it is their absence that makes the lung look black. Vascular shadows will disappear if the lung is replaced by air, which will occur with a pneumothorax or bullous or cystic lung disease or if the vessels are deprived of blood as in a pulmonary embolus. Therefore think pneumothorax, bullae/cyst or pulmonary embolism and:

1. Look for a lung edge. In a pneumothorax you will see the edge of lung which is not normally seen. Look carefully at the upper zone where air will accumulate first. Your eye is trained to see horizontal lines better than vertical so it is sometimes easier to detect the lung edge with the X-ray turned on its side.

2. Look at the mediastinum. Obvious mediastinal shift away from the black lung suggests that a tension pneumothorax is developing. This is a medical emergency and you need to urgently reassess the patient (see also p. 112).

3. Look at the rest of the lungs. Bullous disease is more likely if bullae or emphysematous changes are seen in the rest of the lung.

4. Differentiating between a pneumothorax and a bulla can be difficult and often impossible. Look at the distribution of the blackness. In a pneumothorax it will be peripheral and upper zone, or lateral and even underneath the lung. Bullae are within the lung and have curvilinear convex margins. In a pneumothorax the edge of the blackness will run parallel to the chest wall, which will not be the case with a bulla lying within the lung.

5. Look carefully for lung markings. If you see them crossing the area of blackness, you are probably looking at a bulla. If you see lung markings peripheral to the blackness, it is also probably a bulla.

Some causes of a pneumothorax

Spontaneous
Iatrogenic/trauma, e.g. pleural tap, transbronchial biopsy, central venous line insertion, mechanical ventilation
Obstructive lung disease, e.g. asthma, COPD
Infection, e.g. pneumonia, tuberculosis
Cystic fibrosis
Connective tissue disorders, e.g. Marfan's, Ehlers–Danlos

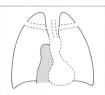

5.3 Tension pneumothorax

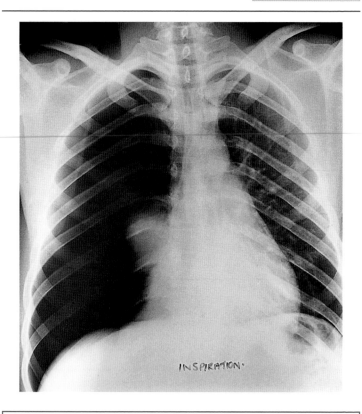

INSPIRATION.

This chest film shows the potentially fatal condition of a tension pneumothorax. The build-up of pressure in the thorax on the side of the air leak can obstruct cardiac venous return. This can be potentially fatal if the pleural cavity is not urgently drained.

If you suspect a pneumothorax as a cause of a black lung field (see p. 110) you must consider carefully whether it may be under tension since this is a medical emergency.

1. Look at the size of the blackness. In a tension pneumothorax the black lung is usually very large.

2. Look at the position of the mediastinum. In a tension pneumothorax it will be shifted away from the affected lung.

3. Look at the shape of the mediastinum. Look at the edge on the side of the blackness. If it is concave to the side of the blackness you should suspect a tension pneumothorax.

4. Always remember the patient. A tension pneumothorax can develop at any time and if the patient suddenly becomes distressed the absence of tension on a previous X-ray does not exclude the diagnosis.

5.4 Pulmonary embolus (PE)

A large pulmonary embolus is a cause of black lung. However, a pulmonary embolism is very rarely detected on a plain chest X-ray and the main reason for doing a plain film is to exclude other causes of shortness of breath, such as pneumonia or pulmonary oedema. Of far more use for the detection of pulmonary emboli are ventilation/perfusion ($\dot{V}/\dot{Q}$) scanning and CT pulmonary angiogram (CTPA).

$\dot{V}/\dot{Q}$ scanning

The $\dot{V}/\dot{Q}$ scan is a nuclear medicine test. This uses small low-dose radioactive particles to compare the pattern of perfusion with that of ventilation. For the ventilation part of the test the particles are suspended in a gas, which is then inhaled, and stick to the walls of the airways to show airflow. For the perfusion part of the study the particles are injected intravenously and lodge in the very small blood vessels in the lungs. The distribution of radioactivity within the lung is then monitored using a gamma camera. Normally four views are taken (anterior, posterior, and right and left posterior oblique).

In the normal lung ventilation and perfusion should match. In a pulmonary embolism the blood supply to a region of lung is reduced but the ventilation maintained, so-called 'ventilation/perfusion mismatch'. In some lung diseases, e.g. pneumonia, the ventilation and perfusion may both be reduced giving a so-called 'matched defect'. Other lung diseases, for example COPD, can result in a mismatch between ventilation and perfusion and in practice in a PE it is very common to see a mixture of both matched and mismatched defects. A $\dot{V}/\dot{Q}$ scan is therefore only of value in a patient with otherwise normal lungs.

The $\dot{V}/\dot{Q}$ scan does not give a definite diagnosis of pulmonary embolism (PE). Instead it gives you the probability of the patient having a PE. As such it must be interpreted alongside the clinical situation. A normal scan will virtually exclude a PE, certainly one of clinical significance.

In order to interpret a $\dot{V}/\dot{Q}$ scan:

1. Look at the plain chest X-ray. Abnormalities on the chest X-ray may affect ventilation and perfusion and so may make interpretation of the scan difficult. A scan can be interpreted with much more confidence in the presence of a normal chest X-ray. Someone with multiple areas of lung pathology on their chest film, e.g. consolidation or extensive COPD, is likely to have an inconclusive $\dot{V}/\dot{Q}$ scan, and may be better investigated by CTPA.

2. Look at the perfusion scan (labelled Q). A dark speckled pattern is seen over the well-perfused areas, with under-perfused areas appearing as lighter holes. Compare these areas to the ventilation scan (marked V). If they also appear light then they are classified as matched defects. If ventilation is normal they are classed as mismatched defects.

3. Make sure that you have looked at both lungs. In the presence of a massive PE it is possible for a whole lung to be obliterated on the perfusion scan.

4. The test needs to be carefully interpreted by a radiologist who will determine the number and size of matched and mismatched defects to work out the radiological probability of a PE.

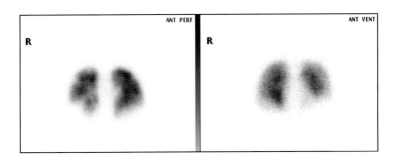

$\dot{V}/\dot{Q}$ scan in patient with pulmonary emboli. Note how the perfusion image is more patchy than the smoother texture of the ventilation scan.

CT pulmonary angiogram

A CT pulmonary angiogram (CTPA) is essentially a contrast enhanced spiral CT scan in which the administration of contrast is timed to high-light the pulmonary arteries. Vessels blocked by clots will appear darker. It is a sensitive means of detecting emboli within central or segmental arteries, although it will not necessarily detect more minor peripheral emboli. Any pulmonary embolus that causes significant breathlessness should be detectable on a CTPA.

Think before you order a CTPA. These scans are often undertaken in young people and involve significant amounts of radiation. Make sure that you have stratified the clinical risk by taking an appropriate history and reviewing the D-dimer result, and consider whether a $\dot{V}/\dot{Q}$ scan or ultrasound imaging of the peripheral veins to look for a deep vein thrombosis would be a reasonable alternative.

In order to interpret a spiral CT scan you need to:

1. Look at the contrast enhanced scans, usually labelled as such.

2. Look at the main pulmonary artery and then follow your way through the scans to examine the major pulmonary vessels. With the spiral CT scan you will be able to visualize the clot, which will appear as a filling defect – a dark area surrounded by whiter contrast. Clot tends to lodge across bifurcations in the vessels and may be seen extending down the vessel towards the periphery. The vessel may be expanded by acute clot compared to the equivalent vessel in the other lung.

3. Look for accompanying features of an embolus. Look on the lung windows for areas of consolidation, which may be wedge shaped, and also look for small pleural effusions.

4. Remember that even if the CTPA does not show a pulmonary embolus it may show another cause for the patient's symptoms.

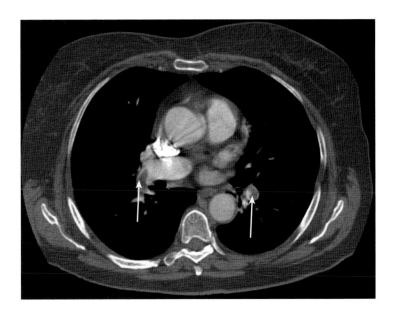

This patient became suddenly short of breath. CTPA showed a pulmonary embolism. Clots can be seen in both the right pulmonary artery and the left lower lobe pulmonary artery. (arrows)

A plain film diagnosis of a pulmonary embolism is very rare.

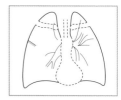

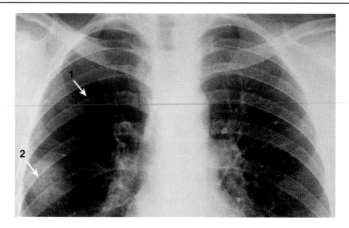

This X-ray is of a patient who has sustained an acute large pulmonary embolus. Look carefully at the right upper zone. Immediately above the horizontal fissure there is an area (1) which is blacker than the left side at the same level. This is Westermark's sign of reduced perfusion to that area of lung which indicates that the artery to this area contains a large clot. Note also an area of consolidation below the horizontal fissure (2) – this is a small focus of infarction.

Changes of infarction

Although a PE is a cause of black lung the findings you will usually see following a PE are those due to subsequent infarction of the lung, leading to haemorrhage or lung necrosis. This may cause the following changes on X-ray:
Raised hemidiaphragm
Collapse and linear atelectasis
Pleural effusion
Wedge-shaped shadowing

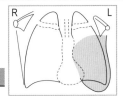

5.5 Mastectomy

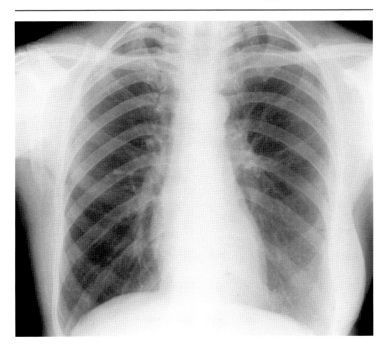

Film of a patient who has undergone a unilateral mastectomy on the right side.

It is important to remember that problems outside the lung can sometimes cause the lung fields to look too black (or too white). This is why it is important always to examine the chest X-ray for soft tissue markings.

A mastectomy will make the underlying lung look too black since there will be less soft tissue overlying the lungs on the affected side, compared to the normal side. Therefore, if one lung looks blacker than the other, look carefully for the breast shadows. There will be an absent breast shadow on the side of the mastectomy.

CHAPTER 6

The abnormal hilum

6.1 Unilateral hilar enlargement . 122

6.2 Bilateral hilar enlargement . . 126

6.1 Unilateral hilar enlargement

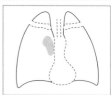

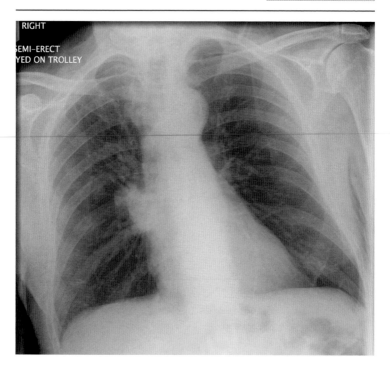

This patient has a bulky right hilum. The contour of the right pulmonary artery is not seen separate to it.

The accompanying CT image shows a lobulated mass lesion at the hilum, and consolidation in the lung posterior to the mass, extending backwards to the chest wall. At bronchoscopy this was shown to be due to a bronchogenic tumour.

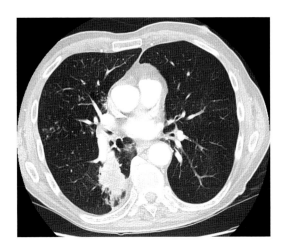

Hilar enlargement is difficult! Suspect unilateral hilar enlargement if:

1. One hilum is bigger than the other (obviously – they should be the same size!).

2. One hilum is denser than the other.

3. There is a loss of the normal concave shape – the hila are usually concave in shape. This concavity may disappear and be the first sign of hilar enlargement.

If you suspect unilateral hilar enlargement then:

1. Check the technical quality of the film. A rotated film will make one hilum appear larger than another.

2. Look at the lateral film. An enlarged hilum may look abnormally dense on the lateral and sometimes this is easier to spot than on the PA.

3. Look at the old films. You will be less worried if the X-ray looked the same 15 years ago!

Now you need to decide whether the enlargement is due to enlarged vascular shadows or enlargement of the hilar lymph nodes or whether it is due to a central bronchial carcinoma superimposed over the hilar shadow. These are the likely possibilities.

1. Look at the edge of the hilum. Vascular margins are usually smooth in nature. Lymphadenopathy gives a smooth lobular appearance. Spiculated, irregular or indistinct margins suggest malignancy.

2. Look for the presence of calcium which will appear as a very dense white. Its presence suggests lymphadenopathy.

3. Look at the rest of the X-ray. If you suspect hilar enlargement then look carefully at the periphery for lung lesions (tumour, TB), lung infiltration (carcinomatous lymphangitis) or bone lesions (metastases).

4. Look at the rest of the mediastinum. Malignant hilar enlargement may be associated with superior mediastinal lymphadenopathy.

Hilar enlargement always warrants further investigation.

Causes of hilar lymphadenopathy

Neoplastic, e.g. spread from bronchial carcinoma, primary lymphoma
Infective, e.g. tuberculosis
Sarcoidosis (rarely unilateral)

Causes of hilar vascular enlargement

Pulmonary artery aneurysm
Post-stenotic dilatation of the pulmonary artery

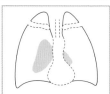

6.2 Bilateral hilar enlargement

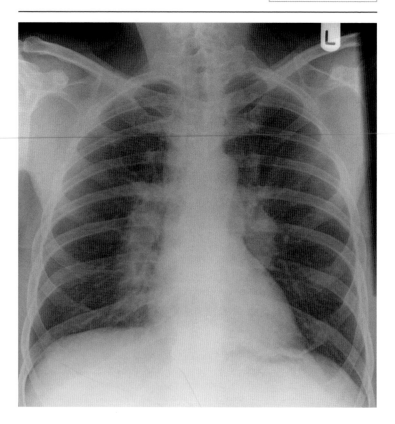

In this patient both hilar regions are enlarged. The pulmonary arteries leading away from the hila are normal in size. This indicates that there is lymph node enlargement at both hila. This patient was a 30-year-old man with a skin rash, erythema nodosum, and his diagnosis was sarcoidosis.

As with unilateral hilar enlargement, bilateral hilar enlargement can be due to enlargement of pulmonary arteries, veins or lymph nodes. The features that suggest hilar enlargement are described on page 123. In bilateral enlargement they are present on both sides! The commonest causes of bilateral hilar enlargement are pulmonary hypertension and sarcoidosis. You should start off by looking for features of either of these. If you suspect pulmonary hypertension then:

1. Look at the periphery of the X-ray. Pulmonary hypertension is associated with peripheral pruning which means that the blood vessels appear cut off before they reach the outer $\frac{1}{3}$ of the lung. The edge of the lung fields are, therefore, often darker than usual and the central area often whiter.

2. Look at the shape of the hila and lower lobe pulmonary arteries. The lower lobe pulmonary arteries will also be big in pulmonary hypertension but of normal size if hilar enlargement is due to lymphadenopathy. The hila are, therefore, convex in shape in pulmonary hypertension.

3. Look for a cause of pulmonary hypertension. Look for signs of lung disease such as COPD and look carefully at the shape of the heart for chamber enlargement, for signs of left to right shunts or mitral stenosis.

If you suspect sarcoidosis then enlargement of the hilum may be the only finding. However, other features are often present and you should look for:

1. *Small nodules.* These are between 1.5 and 3 mm in diameter, are mostly found in the perihilar and mid zones, are non-uniform in character, moderately well defined and usually bilateral.

2. *Large nodules.* These are about 1 cm in diameter, have an ill-defined edge and sometimes coalesce to give larger opacities which may contain air bronchograms.

3. *Lines.* The X-ray may demonstrate a network of fine lines emanating from the hilar region.

4. *Honeycombing.* Features of fibrosis may be apparent. Look for these particularly in the upper zones where they are especially common.

Causes of bilateral hilar lymphadenopathy

Sarcoid
Tumours, e.g. lymphoma, bronchial carcinoma, metastatic tumours
Infection, e.g. tuberculosis, recurrent chest infections, AIDS
Berylliosis

Causes of pulmonary hypertension

Obstructive lung disease, e.g. asthma, COPD
Left heart disease, e.g. mitral stenosis, left ventricular failure
Left to right shunts, e.g. atrial septal defect, ventricular septal defect
Recurrent pulmonary emboli
Primary pulmonary hypertension

CHAPTER 7

The abnormal heart shadow

7.1 Atrial septal defect. 130
7.2 Mitral stenosis 132
7.3 Left ventricular aneurysm . . .134
7.4 Pericardial effusion 136

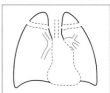

7.1 Atrial septal defect (ASD)

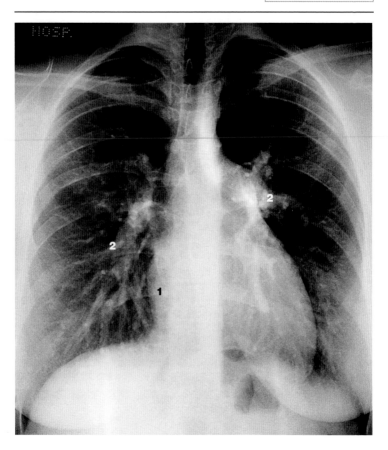

This X-ray shows the typical appearance of an atrial septal defect. The heart is enlarged, the apex is rounded, the right atrium prominent (1) and the pulmonary arteries are dilated (2) due to increased pulmonary blood flow.

Always remember to study the heart and the pulmonary arteries. If the heart is enlarged or pulmonary hypertension is present then one possible cause is an ASD. If you suspect an ASD then look for the following:

1. The heart may be enlarged. Determine the cardiothoracic ratio by measuring the width of the thorax and the width of the heart. If the heart is more than half the diameter of the thorax it is enlarged.

2. Look at the shape of the heart. Look first at the apex which is often rounded due to enlargement of the right ventricle and is sometimes lifted clear of the diaphragm. Next look at the right heart border. Because the right atrium enlarges, the right heart border looks much fuller than normal.

3. Look at the position of the heart by comparing it to the position of the vertebrae. With an ASD the heart is sometimes shifted to the left and so the right edge of the vertebral column is revealed.

4. Look at the aortic knuckle and arch of the aorta. It is often smaller if an ASD is present since blood is diverted to the right atrium rather than passing through the aorta.

5. Check for the signs of pulmonary hypertension (Chapter 6.2).

An ASD is difficult to distinguish radiologically from other left to right shunts. Echocardiography is the most appropriate means of making a diagnosis.

7.2 Mitral stenosis

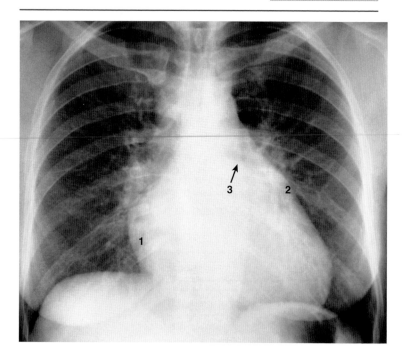

This film is that of a patient who had rheumatic fever when younger. The cardiac contour is abnormal with bulging on the right giving a double right heart border (1), prominence of the left atrial appendage (2) and elevation of the left main bronchus (3), indicating left atrial enlargement. The left atrial pressure is elevated producing increased pulmonary venous pressure with upper lobe diversion (prominence of the upper lobe veins) and basal septal lines of interstitial oedema (see Chapter 4.11).

Mitral stenosis can cause changes in both the shape and size of the heart. It is a cause of pulmonary oedema. If you suspect mitral stenosis:

1. Look at the left heart border. Look just below the left hilum where the border of the heart is made up of the left atrium (Chapter 2.2). This area is usually concave in shape but in mitral stenosis the left atrium is enlarged causing a loss of this concavity and a straightening of the left heart border. Sometimes atrial enlargement is so great that this part of the heart bulges outwards.

2. Look at the right heart border. Look carefully for a double shadow which you sometimes see in a well-penetrated film and is due to left atrial dilatation.

3. Identify the trachea and follow it down until you see it split into right and left bronchi. This is the carina, and the angle between the bronchi should be less than 90°. Measure this angle. If it is more than 90° this may indicate left atrial enlargement, a feature of mitral stenosis. However, there is wide normal variation.

4. Look in the area of the mitral valve for signs of calcification, i.e. flecks of dense white around the valve. This would suggest mitral valve disease, but is a rare finding.

Causes of mitral stenosis

Congenital
Rheumatic fever

7.3 Left ventricular aneurysm

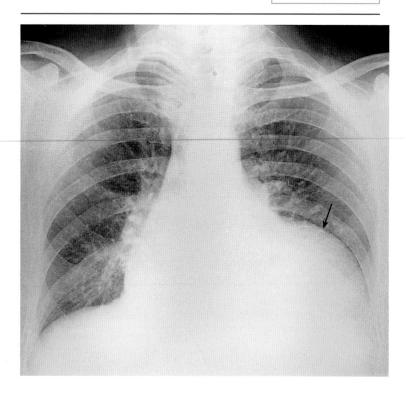

This film is of a 57-year-old man with chest pain and shortness of breath. In addition to the signs of early pulmonary oedema the film also shows a left ventricular aneurysm with an outward and upward bulge of the left ventricular apex. Calcification is also apparent (arrow).

A left ventricular aneurysm is a cause of cardiac enlargement on the chest X-ray. It can often cause generalized enlargement of the left ventricle and be indistinguishable from left ventricular dilatation. If you suspect an aneurysm then look for:

1. A bulge in the left ventricle. Follow the left border of the heart. If a part bulges out then this is suggestive of an aneurysm.

2. Look for calcification. If the aneurysm is longstanding then it may have become calcified and you will see a rim of calcification along the heart border.

Cardiac-related calcification

A left ventricular aneurysm is not the only cause of calcification within or around the heart. Calcification of the pericardium can occur as a result of TB, or asbestos-related pleural plaques on the mediastinal surface. Uraemic pericarditis may also calcify. Often no cause can be found.

7.4 Pericardial effusion

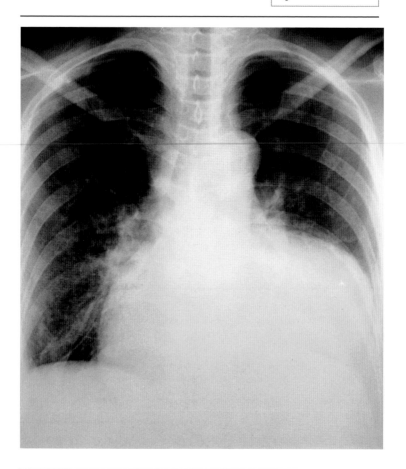

This film shows a pericardial effusion. The heart shadow is enlarged and globular in shape and covers both hila.

A pericardial effusion is another cause of an enlarged heart shadow. If you suspect it then:

1. Confirm that the heart shadow is enlarged. Check that it is a PA film and that the largest diameter of the heart shadow is more than half the largest diameter of the thorax.

2. Look carefully at the shape of the heart shadow. Enlargement due to an effusion is generalized, so if the enlargement appears to be due to a specific chamber enlarging then the cause is unlikely to be an effusion. The heart shadow is globular in shape if an effusion is present, though do not be put off by a bulge that you can sometimes see on the left heart border.

3. Look at the lung fields. If cardiac enlargement is due to left ventricular failure then the vascular markings should be increased making the lung fields whiter than usual. In a pericardial effusion the vascular markings are usually normal.

4. Look at previous films. A sudden increase in heart size is suggestive of a pericardial effusion.

5. Look at the hilum. In a pericardial effusion the heart shadow may cover both hila. This will not occur with other forms of cardiac shadow enlargement.

6. Look at the white line on the edge of the right side of the trachea (the paratracheal density). This should be less than 2–3 mm wide on an *erect* chest X-ray. If it is wider, one cause is enlargement of the superior vena cava. This would be consistent with a pericardial effusion (see also p. 141).

Causes of pericardial effusions

Transudate
  Congestive cardiac failure
Exudate
  Post myocardial infarction
  Infection, e.g. tuberculosis, bacterial
  Neoplastic infiltration
  Collagen vascular, e.g. rheumatoid arthritis, SLE
  Iatrogenic, e.g. post cardiac surgery
  Endocrine – myxoedema
Blood
  Trauma
  Neoplastic infiltration
  Aortic dissection/penetrating peptic ulcer
  Bleeding diathesis, e.g. anticoagulation, leukaemia

CHAPTER 8

The widened mediastinum

The widened mediastinum 140

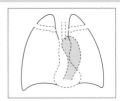

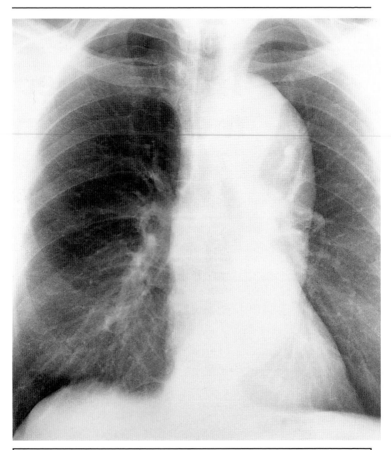

This is the film of a patient with a descending thoracic aortic aneurysm. The mediastinum is widened to the left of the midline throughout its length, with increased convexity around the aortic arch.

Always look carefully at the mediastinum. If you think that it is widened then relate this finding to the clinical history. Try to find some old films and see if the mediastinum has got larger. Be aware that a normal chest X-ray does not exclude a significant aortic event, such as a dissection, and in the presence of clinical suspicion an urgent CT may be an appropriate investigation.

Important causes of a widened mediastinum are thyroid enlargement, enlargement of mediastinal lymph nodes, aortic dilatation, dilatation of the oesophagus or thymic tumours. In deciding a likely cause, go through the following process:

1. Check the rotation of the film. A badly rotated film can make the mediastinum appear widened.

2. Decide whether the enlargement is at the top, middle or bottom of the mediastinum. If at the top it is likely to be thyroid, thymus or innominate artery. If in the middle or bottom of the mediastinum it could be lymphadenopathy, aortic widening, dilatation of the oesophagus or a hiatal hernia.

3. If the shadowing is at the top then look at the position of the trachea. An enlarged thyroid will displace or narrow the trachea. This will not happen with a tortuous innominate artery – a common finding in the elderly.

4. Look at the right side of the trachea. The white edge of the trachea should be less than 2–3 mm wide on an *erect* film. An increase in its width suggests either an enlarged superior vena cava or a paratracheal mass. This rule does not apply to supine films.

5. If you suspect an enlarged thyroid then look at the outline of the shadow. A thyroid has a well-defined outline that tends to become less clear as one moves up the neck.

6. If you suspect widening of the aorta then try and follow its outline, remembering that the root of the aorta is not visible. You may be able to detect a continuous edge which widens to form the edge of the enlarged mediastinum. This would suggest that the widening is due to dilatation of the aorta.

7. The commonest cause of an abnormal whiteness of the mediastinum in the elderly will be unfolding of the aorta. You may be able to trace the margin of the ascending aorta around the arch and to the descending aorta. Some calcification in the wall of the aortic knuckle is a common feature. If the line of calcium is separated from the edge of the aortic shadow this strongly suggests a dissection.

8. A widened, aneurysmal, aorta can sometimes be difficult to distinguish from the more common unfolded aorta. If you can follow both edges of the aorta and detect a widening this suggests an aneurysm. CT is often used to assess aortic dimensions.

CHAPTER 9

Abnormal ribs

9.1 Rib fractures. 144
9.2 Metastatic deposits 146

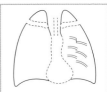

9.1 Rib fractures

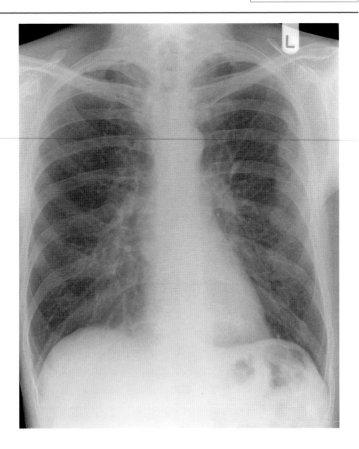

Note how there is increased whiteness over the left side of the chest. On close inspection you can see that the posterior ribs have a step in their alignment – these are fractures affecting the 5th, 6th, 7th and 8th ribs.

Your examination of the chest X-ray is not completed until you have looked carefully at the ribs. They should be of a uniform density with smoothish, unbroken edges. The main abnormalities to look for are old and new fractures and metastases.

1. *New fractures*. Look along the edges of each rib. A new fracture will be seen as a break in the edge. Once you have spotted a fracture look for more information. Look at the position of the fracture. A fracture of any of the first three ribs is unusual and implies tremendous force. Look for other fractures. A line of fractures suggests a traumatic injury whereas fractures scattered throughout the ribs may suggest repeated injury (as in an alcoholic) or underlying bony weakness (as in malignant disease). Look at the density of the ribs and compare them in your mind to other X-rays you have seen. If the ribs are less white than usual this suggests underlying decrease in bone density. Finally look for the complications of rib fractures – surgical emphysema, pneumothorax and haemothorax. Remember also that damage to the lower three ribs may result in hepatic, splenic or renal injury.

2. *Old fractures*. Again look along the edges. The callus formation that follows a fracture will cause the rib to expand at this point. You need to look carefully – sometimes callus formation can simulate a lung mass.

Diagnosis of rib fractures

Rib fractures can be missed on a chest X-ray. The diagnosis is therefore clinical and the chest X-ray is usually performed to look for potential complications.

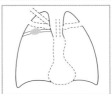

9.2 Metastatic deposits

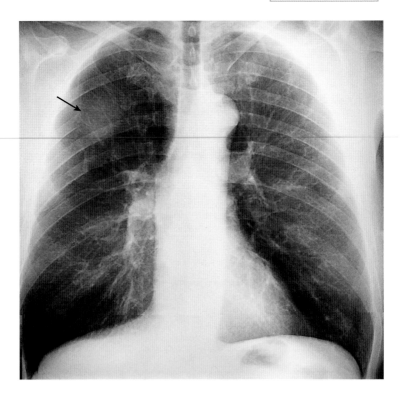

Look carefully at this film. The lungs are overexpanded. Note the destruction of the posterior part of the cortex and the medulla of the right 5th rib with an associated ill-defined soft tissue mass (arrow). This is a lytic metastasis.

Metastatic lesions in the ribs will tend to look like dark holes. Scan the ribs carefully for evidence of metastasis. Secondaries start in the medulla and spread outwards with very little reaction around them so you are literally just looking for a dark hole. Sometimes the underlying lung markings create the impression of a metastasis in the overlying rib. If you spot a dark hole in the rib then look carefully at its edge. Compare the outline to the underlying lung markings. If they overlap then the metastasis may be deceptive. If you see bone metastases check carefully to see whether there is an associated fracture.

Look carefully at the other bones, which may contain similar pathology.

CHAPTER 10

Abnormal soft tissues

Surgical emphysema 150

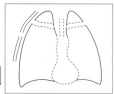

Surgical emphysema

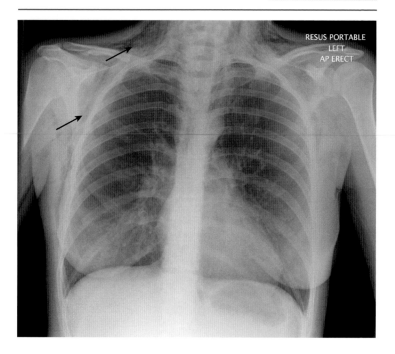

RESUS PORTABLE
LEFT
AP ERECT

This is the film of a young asthmatic patient who presented with chest pain. The film was taken to look for complications of asthma such as a pneumothorax or air in the mediastinum – pneumomediastinum. Neither can be seen, but there is extensive air in the soft tissues (arrows) over her shoulders and along the right chest wall, best seen in the axillary area. There probably is a small pneumothorax, but this cannot be seen on the film.

At first sight surgical emphysema gives a very messy appearance which is sometimes confined to the obvious soft tissue areas but may spread over the whole X-ray. If you suspect surgical emphysema look for the following characteristics:

1. In mild cases look for lozenge-shaped areas of blackness which represent pockets of air in the soft tissue. These areas will all lie in the same plane which will follow the plane of the soft tissue structures.

2. In severe cases the orientation of the planes is lost. Instead look for alternating dark and white lines which appear not to be confined to single structures and cross part or all of the film.

Causes of surgical emphysema

Trauma
Iatrogenic, e.g. surgery, chest drain insertion
Obstructive lung disease, e.g. asthma
Oesophageal injury
Gas gangrene

CHAPTER 11

The hidden abnormality

11.1 Pancoast's tumour 154
11.2 Hiatus hernia 156
11.3 Air under the diaphragm . .158

11.1 Pancoast's tumour

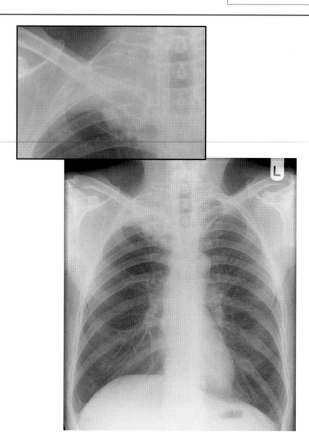

At first glance it may be hard to spot that there is an abnormality on this film. Note, however, the increased whiteness at the right apex. On the magnified image you should also be able to see that the right second rib has fractured – a pathological fracture. This appearance is of a Pancoast's tumour with invasion into the chest wall.

A number of abnormalities can be easily missed. Before deciding an X-ray is normal:

1. Look carefully at the apices of both lungs. This is a common site for lung pathology, for example a Pancoast's tumour or chronic fibrosis. Lesions here can be easily missed because the apex of the lung is hidden by ribs and clavicles.

2. Look carefully at the heart shadow. Lesions behind the heart are often missed because they are obscured by the whiteness of the heart. Look carefully for any parts of the heart shadow that look whiter than the rest. Look also for the triangular shadow of left lower lobe collapse and other subtle changes such as consolidation behind the heart.

3. Look carefully at the mediastinum. Changes in the shape of the mediastinum can be very subtle.

4. Look at the hilum. Changes in the shape or density of the hilum can be easily missed.

5. Obtain a lateral film – some abnormalities are more obvious on the lateral.

6. Read the radiologist's report!

Exams and the normal X-ray

Spotting the abnormality in an apparently normal chest X-ray is a common question in postgraduate exams. If confronted with such an X-ray, then think of the following possibilities:

Apical shadowing
Left lower lobe collapse
Hiatus hernia (fluid level behind the heart)
Dextrocardia (with the X-ray shown the wrong way around)
Mastectomy
Air under the diaphragm
Small pneumothorax

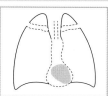

11.2 Hiatus hernia

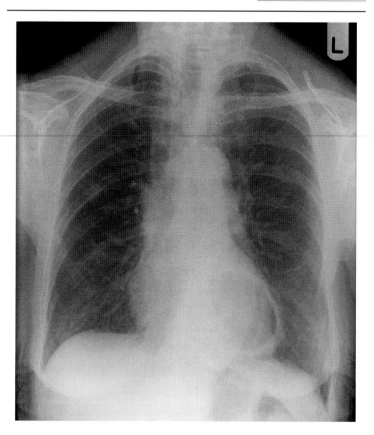

This is the film of a 67-year-old patient who complained of a chronic cough. You can see a curved white line lying behind the heart. This is a hiatus hernia. When questioned, the patient complained of mild heartburn with no other symptoms.

When scanning an apparently normal X-ray it is important to look behind the heart. The heart is usually a fairly uniform white colour and areas of increased whiteness can indicate possible pathology. Therefore if you see an area of increased whiteness behind the heart:

1. Decide whether it has any of the characteristics of the white lung field described previously. For example can you see an air broncho-gram which would suggest consolidation or the tramline or ring-like shadows which would suggest bronchiectasis?

2. Look carefully at the shadowing to see whether it has the appear-ance of left lower lobe collapse. This is described on page 52 and has the appearance of a dense white triangle behind the heart. It is easy to miss so you should look carefully for this.

3. Look to see whether the appearance is consistent with a hiatus hernia. Look for the outline of the stomach which may appear as a rounded white line either behind the heart or next to the left heart border. Look for the flat line of a fluid level which you occasionally see and is caused by fluid within the stomach.

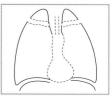

11.3 Air under the diaphragm

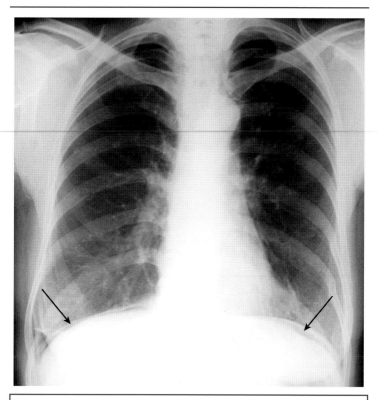

This is the X-ray of a 72-year-old man who presented to casualty acutely unwell with abdominal and chest pain. Examination revealed a silent abdomen. Note the areas of blackness immediately under the diaphragms (arrowed). This represents air collecting under the diaphragm and confirms the clinical suspicion of abdominal perforation. Subsequent history-taking revealed that he had a 2-year history of recurrent upper abdominal pain and on surgery a perforated gastric ulcer was found.

Finish your examination of the chest X-ray by looking at the area under the diaphragm. The area immediately under the diaphragm will usually be white since the upper part of the abdomen contains the dense structures of the liver and spleen. Because of this you can usually only make out the upper surface of the diaphragm. You may see a darker round area under the left hemidiaphragm. This is the air bubble within the stomach.

One of the main reasons for looking under the diaphragm is to detect the presence of free air. This is an important sign since it indicates intra-abdominal perforation. Other intra-abdominal pathologies you might see include areas of calcification (small areas of increased white-ness) under the right diaphragm corresponding to gallstones, and dilated loops of bowel under the left diaphragm.

The chest X-ray is a very sensitive investigation for the detection of free abdominal air since it can detect as little as 10 ml. It appears as a rim of blackness immediately under the diaphragm and you will rec-ognize this since it may enable you to see both the upper and lower surface of the diaphragm.

It is sometimes difficult to differentiate air under the diaphragm from the normal stomach bubble. If in doubt then look at the following:

1. Look at the thickness of the diaphragm, that is the line between the blacker area below and the lungs above. If there is free air immedi-ately below the diaphragm, then the white line between the air and the chest will appear very thin since it will consist of the diaphragm only. If the air is in the stomach then the white line created will consist of both stomach lining and diaphragm and appear thicker. In general, if the line is less than 5 mm, then free air is probably present.

2. Look at the length of the air bubble, that is, the distance from its medial to lateral aspect. If it is longer than half the length of the hemidiaphragm it is likely to be free air, since air within the stomach is restricted by the anatomy of the stomach.

3. Look at both hemidiaphragms. If air is present below the right and left hemidiaphragms, it is likely to be free air in the abdomen.

4. If you are still in doubt order a decubitus film. This is taken with the patient lying on their left side. Free air will rise away from the diaphragm and come to lie lateral to the liver in the uppermost aspect of the abdomen whereas air within the stomach will remain in the same position. Remember that it takes over 10 minutes for these changes to occur so the patient needs to be on their side for 10 minutes before the X-ray is taken.

INDEX

Note: Abbreviations used:
ARDS – adult respiratory distress syndrome
CT – computed tomography

A

abdomen
  perforation, 158, 159
  silent, 158
abnormalities
  classification of, 2
  hidden, causes, 154–5
abscess, pulmonary, 61
acute respiratory distress syndrome
     (ARDS), 85, 86–9
  causes, 88, 89
  complications, 89
  left ventricular failure *vs*, 87
air bronchogram
  ARDS, 87
  lung consolidation, 58, 59,
    60
  lung nodules, 75
  pleural effusion, 66
air bubble
  air under diaphragm, 159
  stomach, 14, 159
airway, mucus plugging, 92–3
allergic bronchopulmonary
     aspergillosis (ABPA), 93
alveolar opacification, in
     ARDS, 87

alveolitis
  cryptogenic fibrosing, 94
  fibrosing, 98
aneurysm, thoracic aortic, 140, 142
angiogram, CT pulmonary (CTPA),
     114, 116–17
anteroposterior (AP) film, 4, 8
aorta
  ascending, CT scan, 32, 33
  descending, CT scan, 32, 33
  dilatation, 141
  tortuous, tracheal shift, 57
  unfolding, mediastinal whiteness,
    141
  widening, 141
aortic aneurysm, thoracic, 140, 142
aortic arch
  atrial septal defect, 131
  thoracic aortic aneurysm, 140
aortic dissection, 141
aortic knuckle, 21
  atrial septal defect, 131
  calcification, 141
aortic valves, prosthetic, 21, 24–5
artefacts, streak, 40
asbestosis, 97
asbestos plaques, 68–9

161

aspergilloma, 80
atelectasis, 93
atrial pacing wire, 22–3
atrial septal defect, 130–1
atrium, left, enlarged, 21, 132, 133

B

bat's wing hilar shadows, 82, 85
'beading,' nodules in sarcoidosis, 97
bones
    metastatic lesions, 147
    scanning on PA film, 12
    see also ribs
brachio-cephalic artery, 30, 31
breath, shortness of, pulmonary embolus, 117
bronchi
    CT scan, 34–8
    in pulmonary fibrosis, 97
bronchial carcinoma
    hilar enlargement and, 123, 124
    lung nodules, 74, 75
bronchiectasis, 90–3, 157
    causes, 93
    high-resolution CT, 91, 92
bronchogenic tumour, 122
bronchogram, air see air bronchogram
bronchopneumonia, 59
bronchoscopy, Pneumocystis carinii (jiroveci) pneumonia, 62
bronchus intermedius, 34
bullae, COPD, 107, 108, 109
bullous lung disease, 111
'bunches of grapes' appearance, bronchiectasis, 90, 91

C

calcification
    aortic knuckle, 141
    cardiac-related, 135
    left ventricular aneurysm, 134, 135
    lung nodules, 75, 101
    mitral valve, 133
    pericardial, 135
    pleural plaques, 69, 72, 73
calcium, unilateral hilar enlargement and, 124
callus, rib fractures, 145
carcinoma see bronchial carcinoma
carcinomatous lymphangitis, 98, 124
cardiothoracic ratio, determining, 131
carina, 133
    angle between bronchi and, 133
    CT scan, 32, 33
carotid artery, 30, 31
cavitation, lung, 78–80
    causes, 81
    nodules, 75
chickenpox pneumonia, 100–1
chronic obstructive pulmonary disease (COPD), 106–9
    CT scan, 109
    V/Q mismatch, 114
    X-ray features, 107–8
cigarette smoking, effect on lung, 109
clavicles, 8
coin lesion, 75, 76
    cavitating, 80, 81
collapse, lung, 42–54
    CT image, left upper lobe, 50, 51
    lateral film, interpretation, 43
    left lower lobe, 52, 53, 157
    left upper lobe, 42, 50, 51
    lingular, 42
    PA film, interpretation, 42
    partial, left, in pneumothorax, 110
    pleural effusion with, 66
    right lower lobe, 42, 48, 49
    right middle lobe, 42, 46, 47
    right upper lobe, 42, 44, 45

tension pneumothorax, 112
volume loss, 43, 54–7, 71
computed tomography (CT)
    scanning, 27–40
  artefacts, 40
  blurring of image, 29, 40
  bronchi, 34, 35, 36, 37
  combined imaging, 29
  COPD, 106, 107, 109
  heart, 32–3, 40
  high-resolution (HRCT) *see* high-
    resolution CT (HRCT)
  interpreting images, 29–40
  interpreting images, scheme for,
    30, 32, 39
  lungs, 32–3
    fissures, 34–8
    left upper lobe collapse, 50, 51
    nodules/coin lesion, 76
    window, 34–8
  lymph nodes, 34–5
  pleural disease, 72–3
  spiral (volumetric, helical,
    contiguous), 28, 29, 34
    pulmonary embolus, 116, 117
  streak artefacts, 40
  trachea, 34–5
  types, 28
  unilateral hilar enlargement,
    123
consolidation, lung, 58–61
  bronchiectasis, 93
  diagnosis, 60
  persistent, 61
  pleural effusion with, 66
  Pneumocystis carinii (jiroveci)
    pneumonia, 63
  pulmonary embolus associated,
    118
  pulmonary fibrosis, 97
contiguous (spiral) CT scan
    see computed tomography
    (CT), spiral

contrast, intravenous, for spiral CT,
    29
costophrenic angles
  pleural effusions, 84, 87
  scanning on PA film, 12
costophrenic sulcus, consolidation
    in, 15
cryptogenic fibrosing alveolitis
    (CFA), 94
CT pulmonary angiogram (CTPA),
    114, 116–17
cystic fibrosis, bronchiectasis,
    93

D

decubitus film, air under diaphragm,
    159
dextrocardia, 8
diaphragmatic tenting, 56
diaphragm(s), 11, 12
  air under, 158–9
  in COPD, 107
  degree of inspiration, assessment,
    9
  identifying on lateral film, 14
  pleural effusions, 66
  pleural plaques on, 69
  scanning on PA film, 11, 12

E

elderly, mediastinal widening,
    141
emergencies
  pneumothorax, 111
  tension pneumothorax, 113
emphysema (COPD), 106, 109
  centrilobular, 109
emphysema, surgical, 150–1
  causes of, 151
empyema, 61, 73
examinations, normal x-ray,
    155

F

fibrosing alveolitis, 98
fibrosis, pulmonary, 94–9
    causes, 97–8, 99
    confirming, 96–7
    consolidation and, 60, 97
    cryptogenic fibrosing alveolitis, 94
    high-resolution CT scan, 95–6
    sarcoidosis and, 97, 98
fissure, horizontal
    checking on lateral film, 14, 19
    lung collapse and, 42, 44, 46
    PA film, 18
fissure, oblique
    identifying on lateral film, 14, 18,
        20
    lung collapse, 43
    lung nodule and, 76
follow-up, lung consolidation, 61
fractures, rib, 144–5
    pathological, 154

G

gastric air bubble, 14, 159
gastric ulcer, 158
glove finger shadows, 91
ground glass density, lung, 97

H

heart
    AP film of, 4, 8
    border, mitral stenosis, 133
    in COPD, 108
    CT scan, 32–3, 40
    lateral film, 21
    left ventricular enlargement, 84
    localizing lesions in, 21–5
    lung collapse film, 42
    LVF see left ventricular failure
        (LVF)
    maximum diameter (PA film), 11,
        84

PA film of, 5
position, atrial septal defect, 131
scanning on PA film, 11
shadow, 9, 11
    abnormal see heart shadow,
        abnormal
    lateral film, 21
    normal, 21, 22, 23
    PA film, 11
shape, atrial septal defect, 131
heart failure
    early signs, 84
    severe, 85
heart shadow, abnormal, 21, 129–38
    atrial septal defect, 130–1
    deviated to side of collapse, 42
    enlarged, pericardial effusion, 137
    hiatus hernia, 159
    left ventricular aneurysm, 134–5
    mitral stenosis, 132–3
    Pancoast's tumour and, 155
    pericardial effusion, 136–8
hemidiaphragms
    degree of inspiration assessment, 9
    see also diaphragm(s)
hiatus hernia, 141, 156–7
    shadowing, 157
high-resolution CT (HRCT), 28–9, 34,
        91
    bronchiectasis, 91, 92, 93
    lung window, 92
    pulmonary fibrosis, 95–6
hilar lymphadenopathy, 124
    bilateral, 98, 127, 128
    causes, 125, 128
    unilateral, 123, 124, 125
hilum, lung
    abnormal, 121–8
    bat's wing shadows, 82, 85
    bilateral enlargement, 104, 126–8
    concavity, 21, 123
    interpreting on lateral film, 14
    loss of concavity, 21, 123

mass, 14, 44
pericardial effusion, 136, 137
pulmonary hypertension causes, 128
right upper lobe collapse, 44
scanning on PA film, 11
unilateral enlargement, 104, 122–5
    diagnostic features, 123
    vascular enlargement causes, 125
'honeycomb' appearance, fibrosis, 94, 95, 96, 97, 127
horizontal fissure *see* fissure, horizontal
hypoxia, *Pneumocystis carinii (jiroveci)* pneumonia, 63

I

infarction, changes of lung, 118
inferior vena cava, CT scan, 32, 33
innominate artery, tortuous, 141
inspiration, degree of, 9
    full, 7
    poor, 6, 9
interpretation, basic (of chest X-rays), 2–3
intra-abdominal perforation, 159

K

Kerley B lines, 84, 85, 87

L

lateral film
    how to look at, 13–15
    localizing heart lesions on, 21, 22, 24
    localizing lung lesions on, 18, 19, 20
    lung collapse on, 43, 48–53 *see also individual conditions*
left atrial enlargement, 21, 132, 133
left atrial pressure, elevated, 132

left ventricular aneurysm, 134–5
left ventricular enlargement, 84, 135
left ventricular failure (LVF), 82–5, 87, 137
    ARDS *vs*, 87
    shadowing, 84
lingular collapse, 42
lobar pneumonia, 58
lobectomy, 56
lungs
    apices of, 66, 155
    asbestos plaques, 68–9
    black field, 105–19
        bilateral, 107
        COPD, 106–9
        unilateral, 110–11
        see also pneumothorax; pulmonary embolus
    borders, of lesions, 20
    bronchopneumonia, 59
    carcinoma, nodules, 74, 75
    cavitating lesions, 75, 78–82
    coin lesions *see* coin lesion
    collapse *see* collapse, lung
    congenital absence (of one), 55
    consolidation, 58–61
    COPD, 108
    CT scan *see* computed tomography (CT) scanning
    empyema, 61, 73
    fibrosis *see* fibrosis, pulmonary
    fields, 11
    fissures
        CT scan, 34–8
        horizontal *see* fissure, horizontal
        oblique *see* fissure, oblique
    ground glass density, 97
    hyperinflation, 54, 146
    hypoplasia, 55
    infarction, 118
    left ventricular failure (LVF), 82–5
    lobar pneumonia, 58
    lobes, CT scan, 34–8

localizing lesions in, 18–20
markings, 108, 111
mesothelioma, 70–1, 72
nodules *see* nodules, lung
opacities, in tuberculosis,
    103–4
overexpanded, 54, 146
pleural effusion *see* pleural
    effusion
pneumothorax, 111, 150
scanning on PA film, 11, 42
size, in fibrosis, 95
tumours, left upper lobe collapse,
    50, 51
upper lobe blood diversion, 84
upper/lower lobe blood vessel
    comparison, 84
volume, *Pneumocystis carinii*
    pneumonia, 63
volume loss, 11, 43, 54–7, 71
white field, 11, 41–104 *see also*
    individual conditions
zones, 20
lung windows, 28
    bronchiectasis, 91, 92
    CT scan, 34–8
lymphadenopathy
    hilar *see* hilar lymphadenopathy
    Pneumocystis carinii (jiroveci)
        pneumonia, 62
    superior mediastinal, 124
lymphangitis carcinomatosis, 98,
    124
lymph nodes
    CT scan, 39–40
    see also lymphadenopathy

M

mastectomy, 119
'matched defect' (V/Q mismatch),
    114
mediastinal window, 28, 30

mediastinum
    abnormal whiteness, 141
    AP film of, 8
    hilar enlargement and, 124
    lymphadenopathy, 98
    miliary shadowing, 104
    Pancoast's tumour, 155
    pneumonectomy and, 55
    pneumothorax, 111
    pulmonary fibrosis, 95, 98
    scanning on PA film, 12
    shift, 64, 66
        pleural effusion, 64, 66
        tension pneumothorax, 113
    tension pneumothorax, 113
    unilateral hilar enlargement,
        124
    widened, 139–42
        causes, 141
mesothelioma, 70–1, 72
metastases, 75, 146–7
    lytic, 146
    miliary, in TB, 103, 104
miliary shadowing, 102–4
mitral stenosis, 132–3
    causes, 133
mitral valves, prosthetic, 21,
    24–5
mucus plugging, of airway, 92–3

N

nodules, lung, 74–7
    air bronchogram, 75
    assessment steps, 75
    calcification, 75
    calcified, causes, 101
    causes, 77
    chickenpox pneumonia, 100, 101
    pulmonary fibrosis, 97, 98, 127
    in right upper lobe, 18, 19
    sarcoidosis, 127
    solitary, 77

O

oesophagus
CT scanning, 32, 33
dilatation, 141
opacities, lung, in tuberculosis, 103–4
orientation, 8

P

Pancoast's tumour, 154–5
paratracheal density, 137
paratracheal mass, 141
penetration, X-ray, 9
peribronchial cuffing, 63
pericardial effusion, 136–8
causes, 138
transudates *vs* exudates, 138
peripheral pruning, in COPD, 108
pleura, 72
increased density, colour, 72
margins, 72
in pulmonary fibrosis, 96
pleural disease, 72–3
CT scan, 72–3
pleural effusion, 14, 64–7, 72, 87
causes, 67
CT scan, 72
large, 64, 72
left, 64
meniscus, 66
in pulmonary oedema, 82
raised hemidiaphragm *vs*, 66
right, 65
simple, CT scan, 72, 73
transudate *vs* exudate, 67
pleural fluid, aspiration/drainage, 66
pleural plaques, 68–9, 72, 73
pleural spaces, in left ventricular failure, 82
pleural thickening, 69, 70, 71
pleural tumours, 71
mesothelioma, 70–1, 72

Pneumocystis carinii (jiroveci)
pneumonia (PCP), 62–3
pneumomediastinum, 150
pneumonectomy, 54, 55
pneumonia, 59
chickenpox, 100–1
lobar, 58
Pneumocystis carinii (jiroveci), 62–3
repeat X-ray and complications, 61
pneumothorax, 110–11, 150
bullous disease *vs*, 111
causes, 111
pulmonary embolus, 114–18
tension, 112–13
diagnostic features, 113
posteroanterior (PA) film, 5, 8, 10
localizing heart lesions on, 21, 22
localizing lung lesions on, 18, 20
lung collapse on, 42, 44, 45, 46, 47
scanning, 2, 10–12 *see also individual conditions*
projection, 8
anteroposterior (AP), 4
posteroanterior (PA) *see* posteroanterior (PA) film
pulmonary abscess, 61
pulmonary angiogram, CT (CTPA), 114, 116–17
pulmonary arteries, 21
in bilateral hilar enlargement, 126, 127
CT scanning, 32, 33
dilated in atrial septal defect, 130, 131
right, in unilateral hilar enlargement, 122
pulmonary embolus (PE), 114–18
CT pulmonary angiogram, 114, 115–16
V/Q mismatch, 114–15, 116
pulmonary fibrosis *see* fibrosis, pulmonary

pulmonary hypertension, 127, 131
  atrial septal defect, 131
  causes, 127, 128
pulmonary oedema, 82, 83, 85
  causes, 87
  left ventricular aneurysm, 134
  mitral stenosis causing, 133
  non-cardiogenic, severe heart
      failure *vs*, 85
pulmonary trunk, 32, 33
pulmonary venous pressure,
      elevated, 132

R

radiologist, 3
respiration *see* inspiration
respiratory failure *see* acute
      respiratory distress syndrome
      (ARDS)
retrosternal space, checking, 14
rheumatic fever, 132, 133
ribs
  abnormal, 144–5
  counting, COPD, 107
  dark holes, metastases, 147
  density, 145
  fractures, 144–5, 154
  metastatic lesions, 147
  pathological fracture, 154
  pneumonectomy and, 54, 55
ring shadows, bronchiectasis, 91
rotation, film, 8

S

sarcoidosis, 97, 98, 103
  bilateral hilar enlargement, 126,
      127
  mediastinal changes, 98
scanning the PA film, 2, 10–12
scapulae, 12
  AP film, 4
  PA film, 5

scoliosis, thoracic, 9
septal lines, 82
  in pulmonary fibrosis, 96
shadow, heart *see* heart, shadow
shadowing, lung, 11
  in ARDS, 87
  basal, 9
  bat's wing hilar, 82, 85
  bronchiectasis, 91, 92
  consolidation and, 60
  glove finger, 91
  ground glass, 97
  left ventricular failure, 84
  miliary, in TB, 102–4
  military, 102–4
  pulmonary fibrosis, 95
  reticular-nodular, 95
  ring, 91
  tramline, 90, 91
  tubular, 91
  vascular, 123–4
silhouette sign, 20
smoking, effect on lung, 109
soft tissue, abnormal, 12, 150–1
stomach
  bubble, 14, 159
  fluid in, 157
streak artefact, CT, 40
subclavian artery, 30, 31
superior vena cava (SVC), 30, 31,
      40
  enlargement, 137, 141
surgical emphysema, 150–1

T

technical quality, 4–9
  checking, 2, 8–9
  interpretation and, 4–8
tension pneumothorax, 112–13
  diagnostic features, 113
thoracic aortic aneurysm, 140,
      142

thorax
    AP film of, 4
    enlarged, COPD, 106, 108
    PA film of, 5
thyroid gland
    CT scan, 30, 31
    enlarged, 57, 104, 141
    mediastinal widening and, 141
trachea
    CT scan, 34, 35
    deviation/shift, 44, 57
    mitral stenosis and, 133
    pericardial effusion, 137
    position, widened mediastinum, 141
    scanning on PA film, 12
tramline shadows, 90, 91
'tree in bud' airway plugging, 93
tuberculosis, 102, 103, 104
tubular shadows, 91
tumours
    cavitating lung lesion, 78
    coin lesion and, 80, 81
    see also bronchial carcinoma

U

upper lobe blood diversion, 84

V

vascular enlargement, hilar, 123, 124
    causes, 125
vascular markings
    COPD, 108
    pericardial effusion, 137
    pulmonary fibrosis, 95
ventilation/perfusion (V/Q)
        mismatch, 114
ventilation/perfusion (V/Q)
        scanning, 114–15, 116
    interpreting, 114–15
ventricular pacing wires, 22–3
vertebral bodies, 52, 53
    checking, 15
    in COPD, 107
    left lower lobe lung collapse, 52, 53
volume loss, lung, 11, 43, 54–7, 71

W

Wegener's granulomatosis, 78
Westermark's sign, 118